Sandplay Therapy

Sandplay therapy: Research and practice explores the essence of sandplay therapy. Drawing on Grace Hong's extensive work in the field, the book discusses this unique, creative and nonverbal approach to therapy. The book focuses on her experiences in practice, research and teaching from both the US and Taiwan.

Divided into five parts and illustrated by in-depth case studies, topics include:

- sandplay therapy research conducted in the US and Taiwan
- the importance of symbols in sandplay therapy
- overcoming depression and trauma through sandplay therapy.

Sandplay therapy: Research and practice will be essential reading for all psychotherapists involved with sandplay therapy, as well as those working with minority groups and those with an interest in cross-cultural psychotherapy.

Grace Hong is a clinical psychologist. She has worked for the Hennepin County Court as a psychologist in the US for thirty years and since returning home to Taiwan in 1999, she has dedicated herself to teaching sandplay therapy in her home country. She is the founding president of Taiwanese Sandplay Therapy Association and works for the Garden of Hope Foundation as an in-house consultant. She is certified in Taiwan and in Minnesota, US as a clinical psychologist and is a teaching member of the International Society of Sandplay Therapy and Sandplay Therapists of America.

Sandplay Therapy

Research and practice

Grace Hong 梁信惠

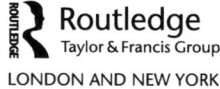
Routledge
Taylor & Francis Group
LONDON AND NEW YORK

First published in Chinese in 2007
by Wu-Nan Publishing Company

First published in the UK in 2011
by Routledge
27 Church Road, Hove, East Sussex BN3 2FA

Simultaneously published in the USA and Canada
by Routledge
711 Third Avenue, New York, NY 10017, USA

Routledge is an imprint of the Taylor & Francis Group, an informa business

© 2011 Grace Hong

Typeset in Times by
RefineCatch Limited, Bungay, Suffolk
Paperback cover design by Andrew Ward

All rights reserved. No part of this book may be reprinted or reproduced or utilized in any form or by any electronic, mechanical, or other means, now known or hereafter invented, including photocopying and recording, or in any information storage or retrieval system, without permission in writing from the publishers.

British Library Cataloguing in Publication Data
A catalogue record for this book is available
from the British Library

Library of Congress Cataloging in Publication Data
Hong, Grace, 1942–
 [Sha you zhi liao yan jiu yu an li. English]
 Sandplay therapy : research and practice / Grace Hong.
  p. cm.
 Includes bibliographical references.
 1. Sandplay—Therapeutic use. I. Title.
 RC489.S25H6613 2010
 616.89'1653—dc22
                                                    2010007263

ISBN 13: 978–0–415–57051–0 (hbk)
ISBN 13: 978–0–415–57052–7 (pbk)

Contents

List of figures	vii
Foreword by Katherine Bradway	ix
Foreword by Chi Hui Jung	xi
Foreword by Barbara Weller	xiii
Acknowledgments	xv
Introduction	1

PART I
Research conducted in the United States   5

1	Introduction	7
2	Literature review	12
3	Method	23
4	Results and discussion	28
5	Conclusion	51

PART II
The author's sandplay case done in the United States   53

6	Introduction of the case	55
7	Zana's sandplay process: recovery from sexual trauma	57
8	Summary	97

PART III
Study of the symbol 101

9 Importance of symbol in sandplay therapy 103

10 Study of the dragon as a symbol 105

PART IV
The author's sandplay research done in Taiwan 115

11 Introduction 117

12 The sandplay outcome study of twelve professional mental health workers 120

PART V
The author's sandplay case done in Taiwan 137

13 Introduction of the case 139

14 Jade's sandplay rebirth process: from darkness to light 141

15 Summary 182

Appendix 186
References 187
Index 191

Figures

7.1	The initial searching	57
7.2	Down to the shadowy land	61
7.3	Grandmother is visiting!	63
7.4	Animals are out	65
7.5	Peace?	67
7.6	A family event	68
7.7	Children, Santa Claus, and animals	70
7.8	Black as a president?	72
7.9	My room	73
7.10	On top of the world	75
7.11	My journey	76
7.12	The demon	77
7.13	The destruction	79
7.14	The wedding	81
7.15	Save the school	82
7.16	They are marrying	84
7.17	Baby on a golden throne	86
7.18	Total death	88
7.19a	Execution	90
7.19b	Execution detail (lower right corner)	91
7.20	Bottom of the ocean	92
7.21	A lively party	94
7.22	Goodbye and thanks	95
12.1	Subject 1's final sand picture	121
12.2	Subject 2's final sand picture	122
12.3	Subject 3's final sand picture	123
12.4a	Subject 4's final sand picture (dry tray)	124
12.4b	Subject 4's final sand picture (wet tray)	124
12.5	Subject 5's final sand picture	125
12.6	Subject 6's final sand picture	126
12.7	Subject 7's final sand picture	127
12.8	Subject 8's final sand picture	128

12.9	Subject 9's final sand picture	129
12.10	Subject 10's final sand picture	130
12.11	Subject 11's final sand picture	131
12.12	Subject 12's final sand picture	132
14.1	The me who is lost	141
14.2	Who is or are under the tombstones?	143
14.3	My tomb	145
14.4	Vast depression and a breathing oasis	147
14.5	Fantasy world	148
14.6	Fireworks of life	150
14.7	The gate	152
14.8	The safe hideout	153
14.9	The flow in front of the rainbow	155
14.10	The spiral	156
14.11	Five islands	158
14.12	A solid fort	160
14.13	After all, I am not an unwanted child!	161
14.14	Mandala	163
14.15	Tears	165
14.16	Four connecting islands	166
14.17	The lonely island	168
14.18	Sea and land	169
14.19	Reappearance of mandala	171
14.20	Peaceful homeland	173
14.21	Almost home!	175
14.22	Going toward the light	176
14.23	Deep and firm blessings	178
14.24	Rebirth	179

Foreword by Katherine Bradway

I was delighted when Grace Hong asked me to write a foreword for her book *Sandplay Therapy—Research and Practice*. This is an important book that will have wide use in the understanding and the teaching and practice of sandplay therapy. The book is divided into five parts: Research conducted in the United States; The author's sandplay case done in the United States; The study of the symbol; The author's sandplay research done in Taiwan; and The author's sandplay case done in Taiwan.

Looking at the chapter headings within each part shows the wide area this book covers in research and practice. The chapters in Part I are: Introduction; Literature review; Method; Results and discussion; and Conclusion. The chapters in Part II are: Introduction of the case; Zana's sandplay process; and Summary. The chapters in Part III are: Importance of symbol in sandplay therapy and study of the dragon as a symbol. The chapters in Part IV are: Introduction and The sandplay outcome study of twelve professional mental health workers. The chapters in Part V are: Introduction of the case; Jade's sandplay rebirth process: From darkness to light; and Summary.

Grace Hong is well qualified to write such a book. Grace has worked for the Hennepin County Court in Minnesota as a court psychologist for thirty years. She graduated from the Minnesota School of Professional Psychology (MSPP) in 1993 and taught one year at MSPP. After her certification in sandplay by STA and becoming a member in STA and ISST in 1996, she then began teaching in Taiwan, her home country. In December 1999, she returned to Taiwan to make her home there and to teach sandplay. She is the only person in Taiwan who is a Teaching Member of ISST and STA. She has served as the first and second-term Chair of the Board since the formation of the Taiwanese Sandplay Association from 2002 till 2008. She also works for the Garden of Hope Foundation as an in-house professional consultant as well as teaching sandplay extensively in Taiwan.

I have known Grace since her days in Minnesota and her activities in the Minnesota Sandplay Society in the mid-1990s. After she returned to Taiwan, we kept in touch with each other through correspondence and personal get-togethers.

The unique feature of this book is that the author, coming from Taiwan and being trained in the US (she has spent about half of her life in Taiwan and half of her life in the US), has the advantage of knowing both cultures thoroughly. In this book, she details her research both in the US and in Taiwan, giving very thorough case studies, one of a Taiwanese woman, and one of an American child. They both overcame the trauma of their lives: the Taiwanese woman felt unwanted as a child, and the American child had suffered severe sexual abuse about three years previously, as well as suffering with periods of severe depression. The American research involved the outcome of twenty sessions of sandplay with ten at-risk children. The psychological test results suggest they became better adjusted, less depressed, more assertive, and have developed better reality-awareness and self-confidence. The Taiwan research had to do with twelve professional sandplay therapists. Their final sand scenes are presented and explained. Their self-reported survey results are presented along with their own views of the process. Finally, the importance of studying the meaning of symbols is presented in the middle part of the book. The study of the dragon is a very good example of knowing the cultural differences in the meaning of symbols and how to do a study of symbols in order to qualify for the certificate in sandplay.

I have always been deeply impressed with Grace's dedication to the practice and research in sandplay. I wrote this foreword for the Taiwanese publication in Chinese of her book. Now I am very happy to know that this book will be published in English and hope that the book will be a useful contribution to English-speaking people.

Katherine Bradway
Founder, STA and ISST
Author, *Sandplay: Silent Workshop of the Psyche*

Foreword by Chi Hui Jung

When someone asked me: "What is sandplay therapy?", I always loved to bring him/her to the sandplay therapy room that is located in the Dandelion Counseling Center of the Garden of Hope Foundation (GOH). In that room, there are shelves equipped with enormous amount of eye-catching miniatures and two sand trays, one wet and one dry. Without any doubt, both visitors and I love to touch the sand and play with the miniatures, reminding me of the unforgettable childhood experience of playing in sand, fun, and touching.

The beginning of sandplay at GOH was initiated by Dr. Grace Hong. She moved back to Taiwan and joined the GOH as a board member and as a professional consultant, greatly helping and impacting the counseling profession in this agency. As the progress that sandplay has made in helping sexually abused clients in this agency, the GOH board has decided to promote sandplay in this agency, to help form the Taiwanese Sandplay Therapy Association, and to help sandplay's promotion in other areas of Taiwan.

Sandplay therapy has a major nonverbal component and is a nontraditional and very creative therapeutic approach. It will bring clients into the unconscious, opening the secret garden of the psyche, and to the shadow that is dreadful for most people to uncover. Therefore it is very challenging to both the therapist and the client. The therapist, in this realm, can become the bridge between the client's conscious and unconscious, the expressed and the hidden, and his/her inner world and his/her outer world.

Sandplay is tremendously powerful; it can heal and it can also destroy. Thus, Dora Kalff, the founder of sandplay therapy, strongly advised sandplay therapists to undergo self-process first and to receive supervision before providing sandplay therapy for clients, regardless of their previous professional backgrounds.

Even though I am not a therapist, I got into the sandplay process because of the need in my work. Just as Jade, the last case in this book, said, "The best accomplishment that I got from completing the sandplay process was the fact that I became in touch with myself; everything is real and sturdy." Through the sandplay process, I obtained a balance of conscious and unconscious;

it was as if I had found the way home. It was truly a beautiful and wonderful process.

I am deeply thankful to Dr. Grace Hong. She has brought sandplay to GOH and to Taiwan. Through her hard work, going to various places in Taiwan to teach and conduct sandplay processes, there are nearly a hundred professionals, including counselors, social workers, psychologists and psychiatrists, who have learned sandplay. It is expected that, in the near future, the seeds of sandplay will flourish in this island, and many of the broken-hearted will be healed.

It is so exciting that after her book *Sandplay therapy: Research and practice* was published in Chinese (by Wu-Nan Publisher) in Taiwan, her book is now published in English. I trust that this book will help, not only those who read Chinese, but also those who are fluent in English, to be more in touch with this mode of therapy either in theory or in practical work and to expand their professional realms. It is my honor to write this foreword.

Chi Hui Jung
Executive Director, Garden of Hope Foundation
Chair, Taiwanese Sandplay Therapy Association

Foreword by Barbara Weller

Two years ago, Grace Hong gave me a copy of her newly published book on sandplay therapy. Much as I looked forward to reading it, I could not—it was written entirely in Chinese. She had written the history of her journey in sandplay, a history of the international society and of our local Minnesota group, about her research project in Minneapolis, her symbol paper, and several case histories; in part, I think, to provide a record of sandplay for her students in Taiwan. Now that the book has been translated into English, I am honored to be asked by Dr. Grace Hong, my former student, and now distinguished teacher, to write the foreword to the English translation of *Sandplay therapy: Research and practice*.

Reading an account of experiences in which one has had a small share is a rather eerie, enlightening, and humbling experience. Eerie, because one has a strange sense of having one's views of events and information adjusted, changed—as if looking through a camera lens at an experience already defined as what one thought was "the way it was" and realizing yet again that fresh eyes, another psyche, and another cultural view of the very same events produces a new and often different focus. Enlightening, because, after years of practice, supervision and teaching, reviewing student papers and discussing their experiences, one becomes aware that there is always new knowledge and fresh ways of looking at information. Humbling, because one comes once again to the realization that no one knows it all, no one has "the right way" of doing or learning something, and that truly, our students *are* our teachers.

Dr. Hong continues describing her journey as she relates her work in Taiwan, organizing a new national society, where she relies heavily on her religious faith to give her the strength and courage to proceed in this heroic task of serving as therapist, then as teacher and supervisor, to over a hundred professional people. She faces the problems of a pioneer when she must wear these different hats in quick succession to achieve the task she has undertaken. As she relates her highly personal journey through the stages of her training, her original paper on a symbol, and the case report which completed the requirements for membership to the International Society for Sandplay

Therapy, it is clear that she then turns quickly to what she sees as her life's work—bringing this therapeutic approach to her home country.

Dr. Hong presents a great deal of raw data in the sections on research and in the cases she presents which can provide rich material for others interested in the research of sandplay as a therapeutic modality. Her symbol paper could be a springboard for other publications as she delves deeper into the meaning of symbols to the eastern, Oriental psyche, compared with the western, Occidental meanings—work which has been begun by some of our sandplay elders such as Dr. Hayao Kawai of Japan. I apologize to Dr. Hong if I appear to be resuming my former role as her teacher, giving her yet another assignment. I offer these suggestions from my eagerness, as one who is learning from her, to ask for "more, more!"

Hanging above my desk is the letter which I received from Dora Kalff, founder of the International Society for Sandplay Therapy, after my submission of a case for final approval as a member of the ISST. In it, she accepts my work, welcomes me to the society, and adds a simple paragraph:

> I hope that in the future you will continue to be actively involved in a process of exchange with other members of the experience you make with Sandplay. This sharing is one of the things that this Society hopes to further.

Grace Hong followed her dream and is bringing sandplay to Taiwan. Her book, in which she shares this experience, is another fulfillment of Dora Kalff's dream for the International Society. Thank you, Grace. Namaste.

Barbara Weller
Certified member of ISST

Acknowledgments

With deep gratitude in my heart, I first thank the Lord, Almighty God, the Father who provides me a spiritual fort, the one who touches my heart, teaches me the truth, and shows me enormous compassion, comfort, and warmth. I truly believe that He is the one who has guided me to the path of psychotherapy and the one who has led me to the sandplay journey. Without Him, I could not have completed the task of publishing my sandplay work that is this book. Thanks to my Lord!

Having said the above, my heart also goes out to many people who have been there for me in this sandplay therapy endeavor, both in the United States and in Taiwan. Introducing me to this wonderful therapeutic approach was my rite-of-passage teacher, therapist, and now friend, Barbara Weller. She has steadfastly supported me in learning, practicing, and teaching sandplay, and this has sustained me during this rather challenging life path. Moreover, many colleagues in the Minnesota Sandplay Therapy Group (MSTG) were there for me during the conduct of the Part I research, Part II case study, and Part III symbol study.

In addition to my MSTG friends, many Sandplay Therapists of America (STA) and International Society for Sandplay Therapy (ISST) members have contributed greatly to my devotion to the teaching and learning of this therapeutic approach. In particular, several of them have been my teachers as well as friends. Katherine Bradway and her husband Brad (now passed away) warmly welcomed me into their house, allowing me to conduct an interview for the benefit of the Taiwanese Sandplay Therapy Association members. Kazuhiko Higuchi came to Taiwan numerous times; he has helped the Taiwanese sandplay community tremendously. The well-respected and beloved Dr. Hayao Kawai, who passed away in 2007, carried out the promise that he made to me (in 2002 at the Japanese Sandplay Conference) by coming to Taiwan in 2004 and teaching sandplay. At that time he still held the post of the Chief of Japanese Cultural Affairs. Together with Dr. Yamanaka and Dr. Higuchi, the three most respected sandplay teachers from Japan provided a sandplay feast for those of us in Taiwan. Martin Kalff, teaching member of ISST and son of Dora Kalff, the sandplay pioneer, came to Taiwan from

Europe in 2006, along with Dr. Higuchi and Dr. Sherry Shepherd from Japan; the three of them conducted workshops for Taiwanese sandplay learners. In 2008, Dr. Rie Rogers Mitchell and Harriet Friedman arrived in Taiwan and lifted the sandplay community enormously. I should add that Gretchen Hegeman and Kate Adams from the US have also contributed to the teaching of sandplay in Taiwan. Without all these colleagues and friends, I could not have accomplished the task of learning and writing about sandplay.

I am most indebted to Chi Hui Jung, the Executive Director of the Garden of Hope Foundation (GOH) and the new Chair of the Taiwanese Sandplay Therapy Association. Upon my return to Taiwan, she invited me to teach sandplay at several locations of the GOH in Taiwan; she graciously provided spaces for me to teach and conduct sandplay processes. The seeds of sandplay, thus, are spread all over this island country; they have sprouted, flourished and grown.

Without any doubt, all the participants in the research that I conducted in the US and in Taiwan were life warriors; they bravely engaged in sandplay processes and graciously consented to release their information. To them, I owe a big thanks. Special thanks to Zana, the 11-year-old Caucasian girl, and Jade, the middle-aged Taiwanese woman. They were my teachers; I learned a lot from them about life and about sandplay therapy.

Most importantly, I am deeply appreciative of all the support and efforts of my family members who have been there with me in this life journey, in the sandplay pursuit, and in this book-publishing process. My husband, David Hong, has always been there for me; he provided me a great deal of freedom to reach for professional growth; he also gave me a warm and loving home. My daughter, Minna Hong, has been most instrumental in the making of this book. She typed, edited, and provided many insightful remarks about my work. She has been a great companion in this book-publishing journey. My son, Steve Hong, a genius in modern technology, has helped me with the editing and arranging of sandplay pictures, and in creating the tables. I am so grateful to you all.

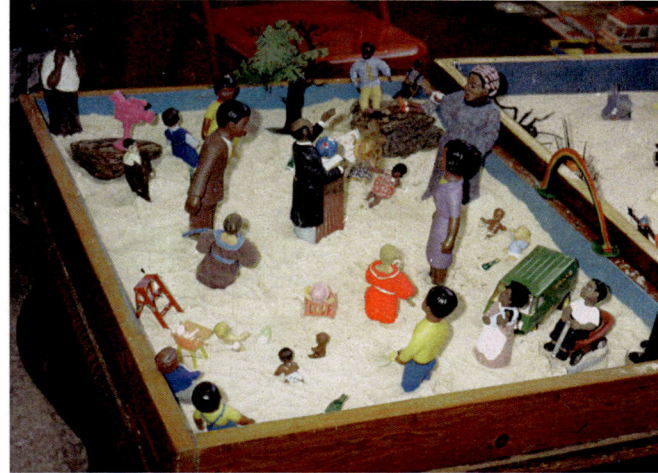

Figure 7.1 The initial searching.

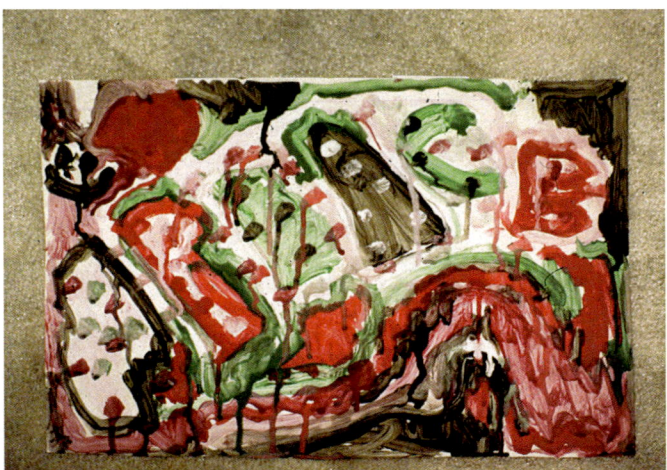

Figure 7.5 Peace?

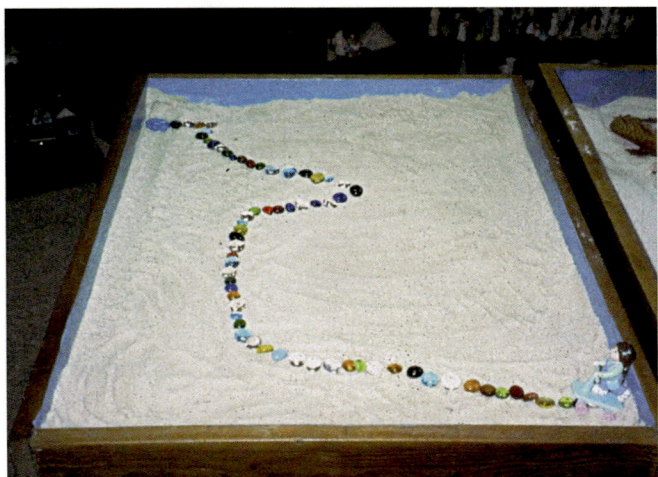

Figure 7.11 My journey.

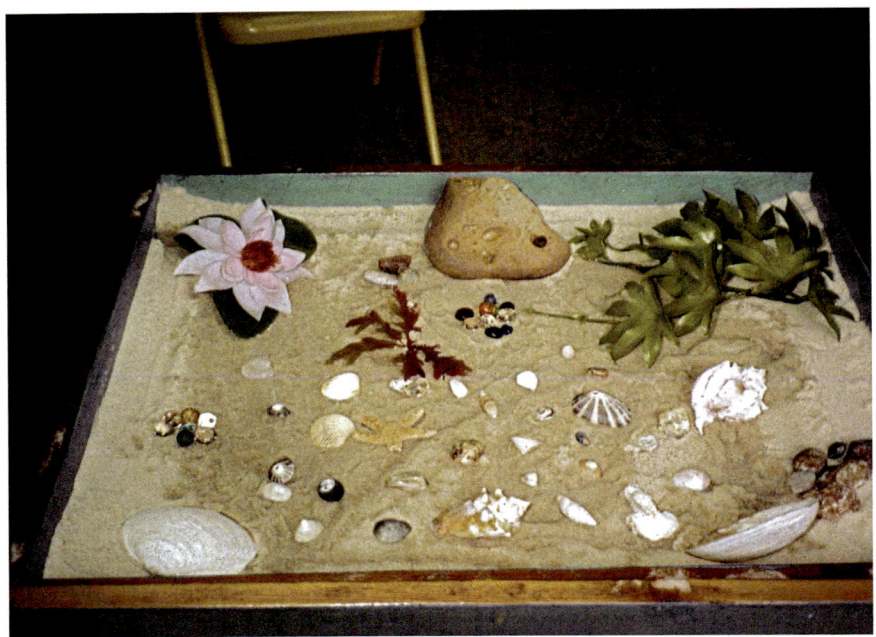

Figure 7.20 Bottom of the ocean.

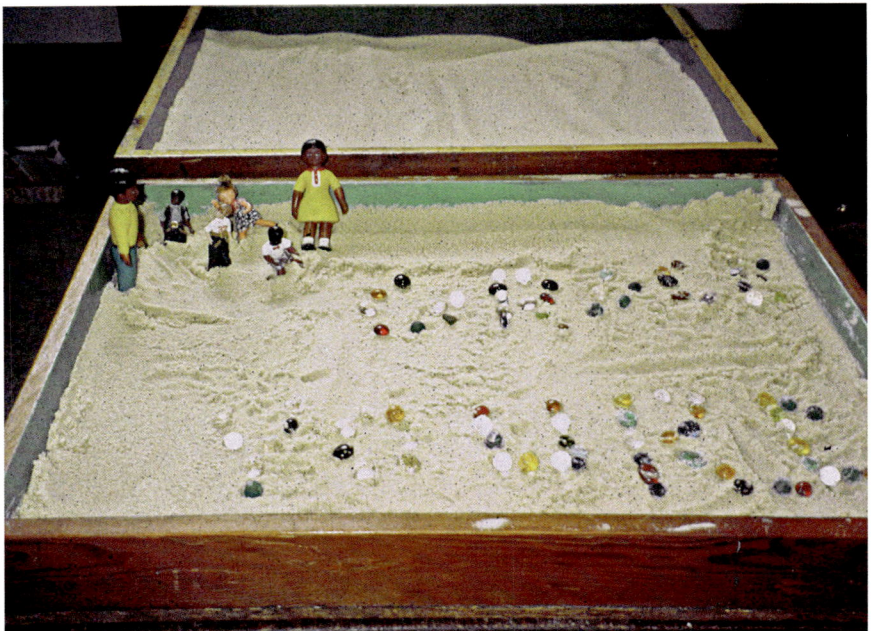

Figure 7.22 Goodbye and thanks.

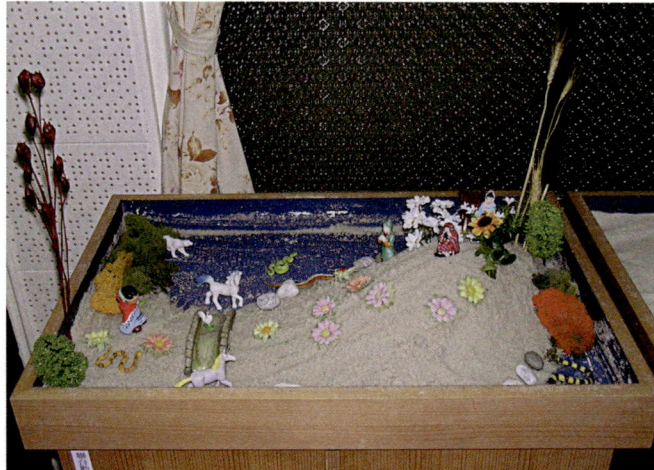

Figure 12.1 Subject 1's final sand picture.

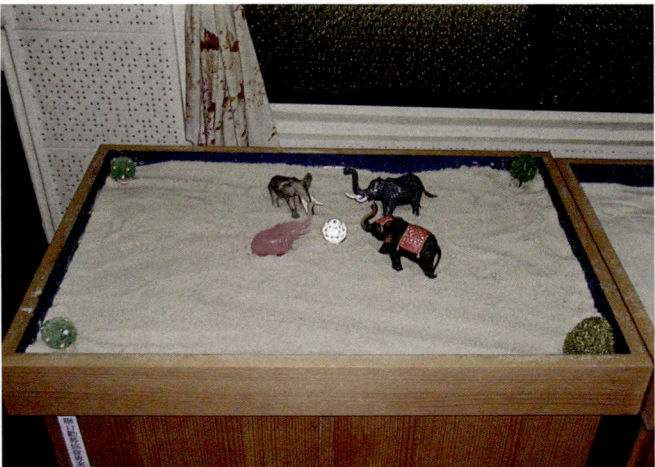

Figure 12.2 Subject 2's final sand picture.

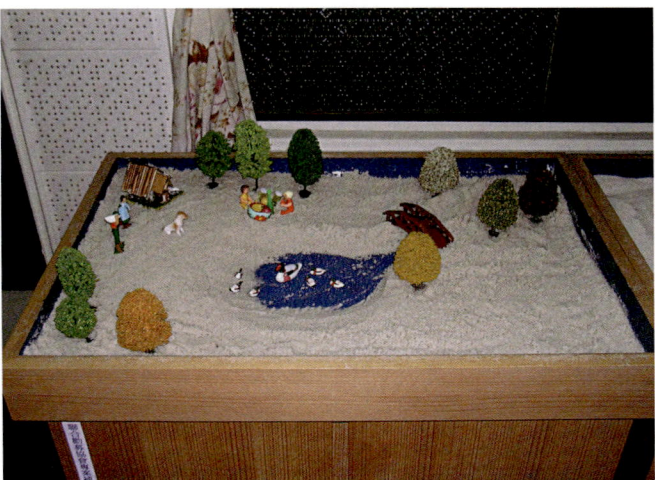

Figure 12.3 Subject 3's final sand picture.

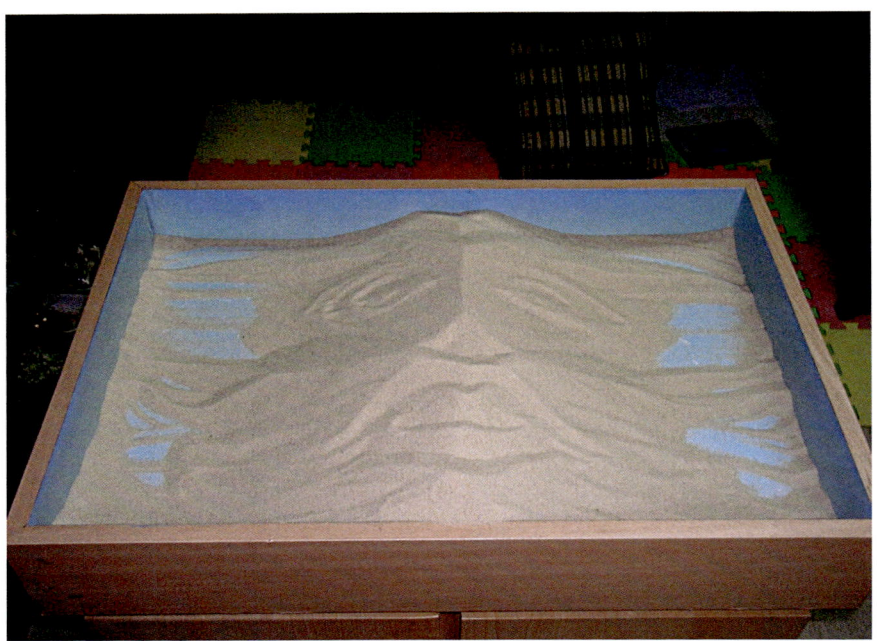

Figure 12.4a Subject 4's final sand picture (dry tray).

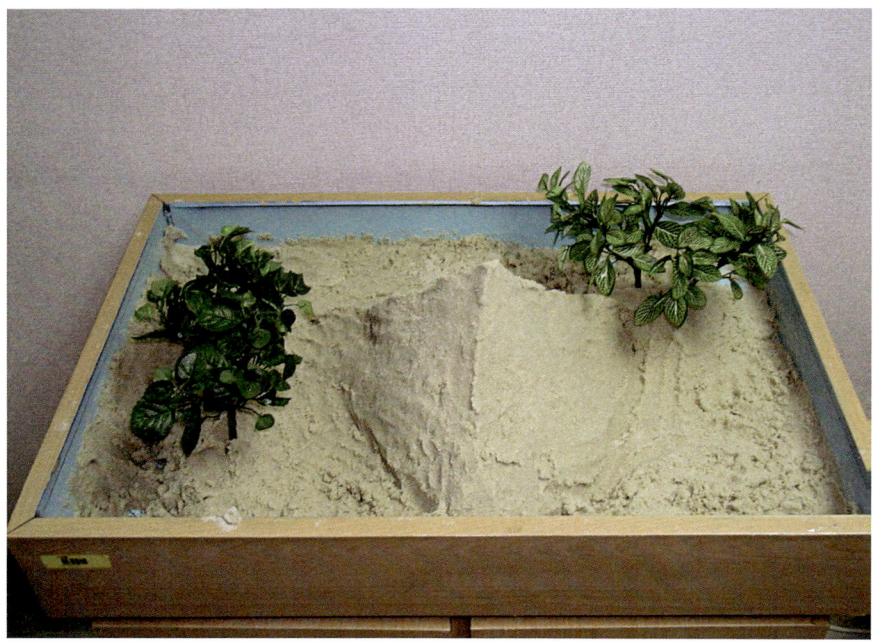

Figure 12.4b Subject 4's final sand picture (wet tray).

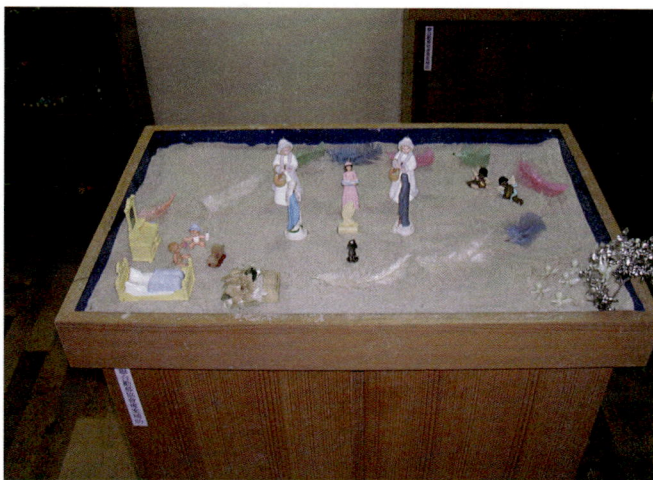

Figure 12.5 Subject 5's final sand picture.

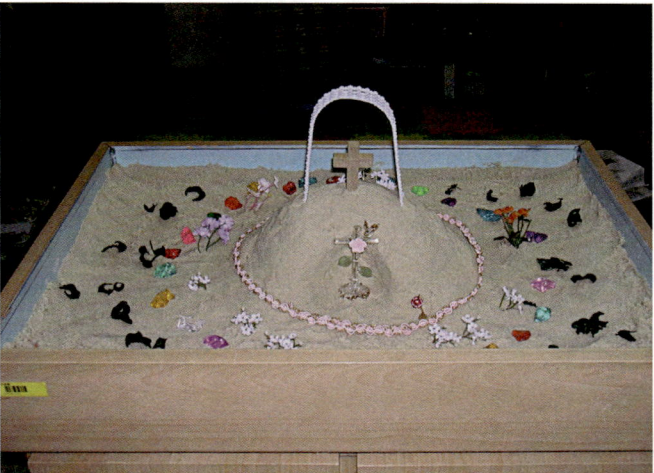

Figure 12.6 Subject 6's final sand picture.

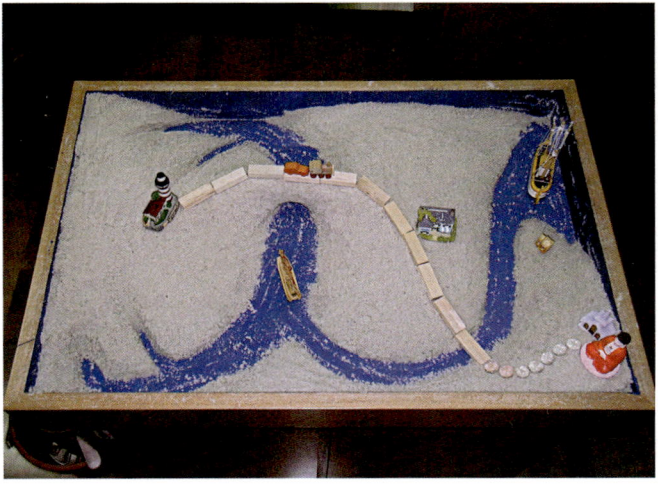

Figure 12.7 Subject 7's final sand picture.

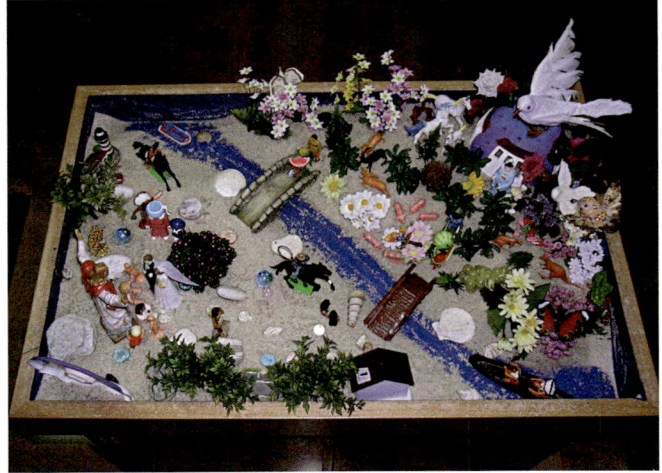

Figure 12.8 Subject 8's final sand picture.

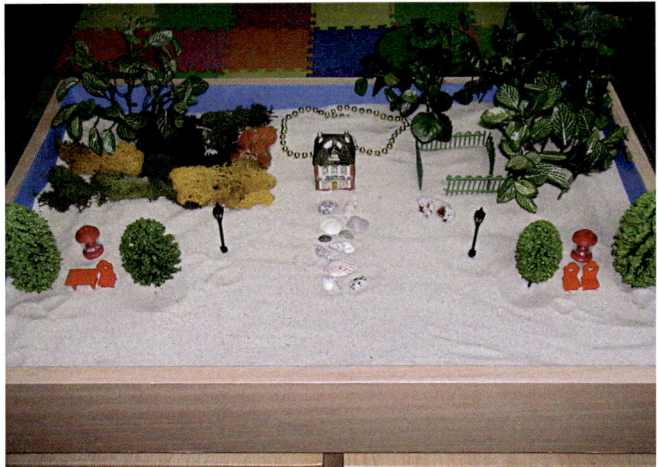

Figure 12.9 Subject 9's final sand picture.

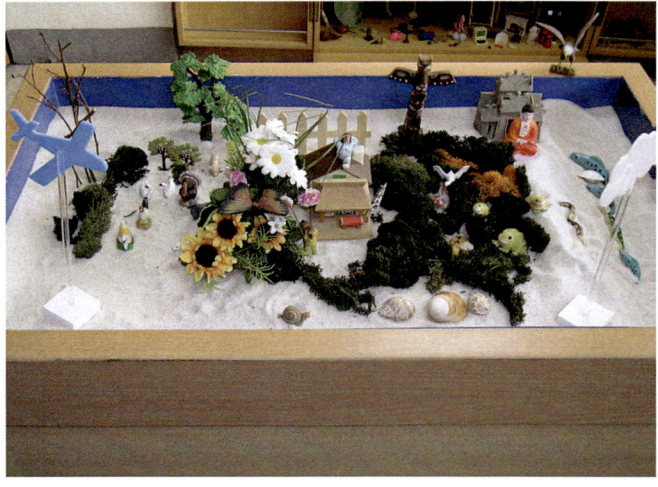

Figure 12.10 Subject 10's final sand picture.

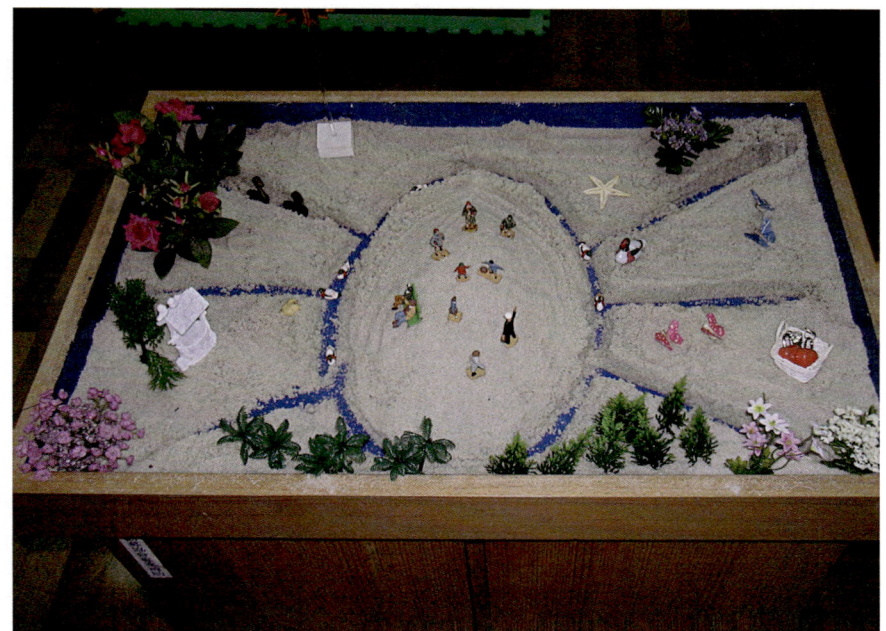

Figure 12.11 Subject 11's final sand picture.

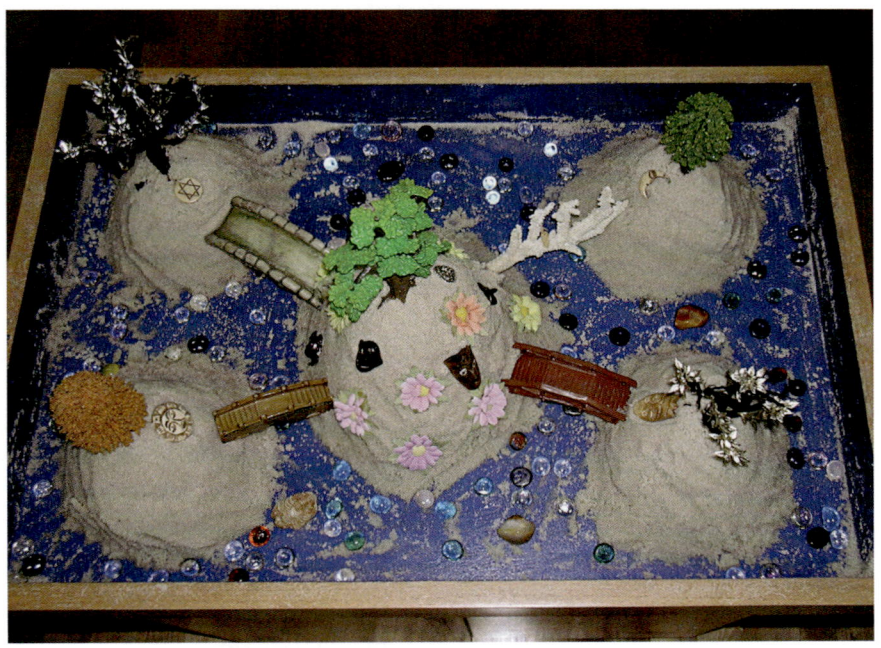

Figure 12.12 Subject 12's final sand picture.

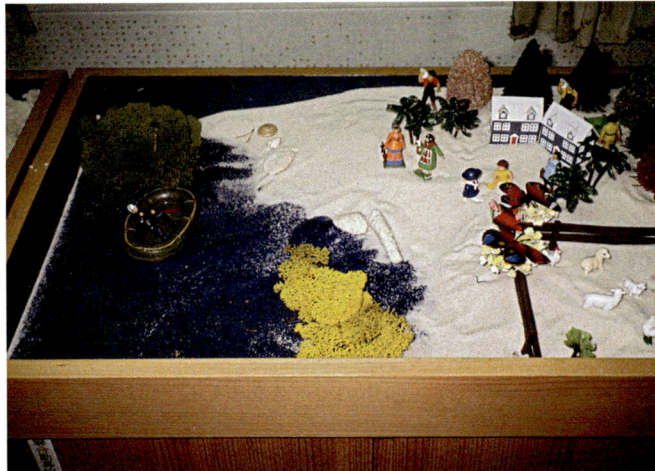

Figure 14.1 The me who is lost.

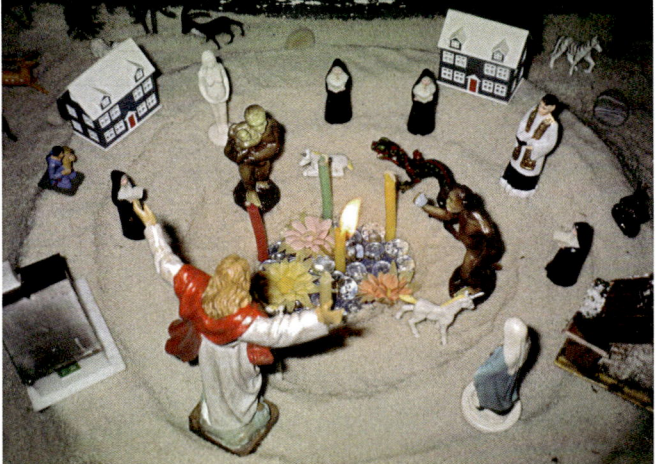

Figure 14.14 Mandala.

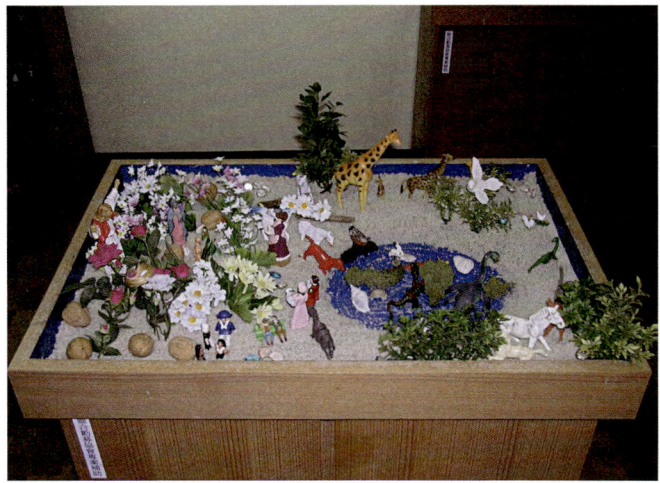

Figure 14.23 Deep and firm blessings.

Introduction

Since the autumn of 1964 when I graduated from the psychology department of the National Taiwan University, I have been working and studying in the clinical psychology field, both in Taiwan and in the United States. It was not until twenty-seven years later that I learned about sandplay therapy. When I first heard about it in the fall of 1991 in a play therapy class at the Minnesota School of Professional Psychology (MSPP), I knew it was in my destiny to learn this unique, creative, nonverbal psychotherapy approach, and to bring it to Taiwan, my home country, to teach and share. With a great deal of determination, effort, and monetary costs, I obtained the certification of Sandplay Therapists of America and the International Society of Sandplay Therapy in 1996.

Near the end of 1999, my dream of returning to my home country, Taiwan, came true. From that time on, I devoted 100 percent of my time to promoting sandplay therapy in Taiwan. With the Lord's blessing, I and several colleagues were able to form the Taiwanese Sandplay Therapy Association in 2002. This association has been instrumental in helping me expand the teaching and practice of sandplay therapy in Taiwan.

In the past eighteen years, my professional life has been primarily focused on learning, studying, teaching, giving sandplay processes, and researching in sandplay. Even though I know my sandplay experiences are not as vast and as extended as those of some of my sandplay colleagues, my dual cultural background of spending half of my life in Eastern Asia and the other half in the United States provides me the benefit or the edge of possessing a wider and more integrated worldview. Thus, I bravely embrace the opportunity to publish my sandplay practice and research in Taiwan and the US for the larger psychotherapy professional society.

Those of us who have been in the field are aware of the fact that it is important to know one's strengths and one's weaknesses. Here I would like to confess that even though I have an advantage of vast clinical experiences, both in the field of psychological assessment and psychotherapy, my weakness is in the area of research. Allow me to partly rationalize this shortcoming to my stubborn insistence on focusing on the client's welfare. However,

I think it is more due to the fact that my artist's nature wins out over my scientist's nature. So, I hope readers will bear with me and forgive me for any imperfection in the research design that I utilized in this book.

There are five parts to this book. The first two parts consist of a research study and a case study that were done in the US, and the last two parts are a research study and a case study that were done in Taiwan. The middle part is a study of the symbol dragon. The research that was done in the US involves ten elementary-school, at-risk children, each of whom had twenty sessions of sandplay therapy, and pre-therapy and post-therapy psychological testing. The tests given were the Children's Depression Inventory, the Rorschach (Exner Method), the Teacher's Report Form, and the House-Tree-Person drawings. Outcome results of the twenty sessions of sandplay therapy for these ten children were analyzed.

The US case involved an 11-year-old Caucasian girl who was sexually abused at an earlier age and who was a subject of the aforementioned research study. Her entire sandplay process has been presented here. It clearly demonstrated her tremendous recovery from the abuse. In contrast, a Taiwanese middle-aged woman's sandplay process showed a miraculous rebirth of this client as she emerged out of a severe depression which involved serious suicidal risk. The latter noted that she felt as if a curse had been lifted off a princess; she became in touch with herself and found her "home."

The research that was done in Taiwan illustrated the outcome of the completed sandplay processes of twelve professional women. In their self-reports, a majority of them (three-quarters) noted that the sandplay processes positively impacted their emotional stability, self-confidence, objective awareness of events in life, psychological energy, and spiritual growth, whereas one-half stated that the gains of the process were in the areas of self-image/concept, interpersonal relationships, problem-solving ability and independence or self-assertion. Improvements in other areas of psychological adjustment were also evident. These participants' final sand pictures show many positive images, including wholeness, serenity, fruitfulness, rebirth, and immortality.

The third part of this book focuses on the study of the symbol that is urgently important for those who are engaging in this therapeutic modality. Using the study of the dragon as a model, we will find out that it is crucially important to learn symbols and to know how to apply them to sandplay therapy. In my teaching, I often was amazed by sandplay students' symbol reports; they inevitably enlarged the narrow conscious view and reached deep into the realm of the unconscious.

Most people who know me well will also know that outside of my extreme devotion to the sandplay practice, my most important commitment lies in the area of my Christian belief. Thus lastly I would like to quote two verses from the Holy Bible to share with readers, and I hope we will be able to heal (bind up) those who are broken-hearted.

The spirit of the Lord God is upon me; because the Lord hath anointed me to preach good tidings unto the meek; he hath sent me to bind up the broken-hearted, to proclaim liberty to the captives, and the opening of the prison to *them that are* bound; To proclaim the acceptable year of the Lord, and the day of vengeance of our God; to comfort all that mourn.

(Isaiah 61:1–2)

Part I

Research conducted in the United States

Chapter 1

Introduction

In the fall of 1991, while I was a student at the Minnesota Professional School of Psychology, I took a course in play therapy. During one particular lecture, my instructor, Dr. Jacquelyn Wiersma, brought in a guest lecturer, Barbara Weller, ACSW, who is one of the founders of the Minnesota Sandplay Therapy Group. I volunteered to help Ms. Weller put up the posters that were part of her presentation. Later, she gave us a brief introduction to sandplay therapy. This proved to be one of the most pivotal events in my life. I began to take more sandplay therapy seminars and workshops. In addition, I started my own sandplay therapy process, and I completed this process in April, 1992. Shortly thereafter, I was given the chance to work on a sandplay therapy project, sponsored by the MSTG. All the therapists who participated in this project were supervised by Barbara Weller, who is a certified member of the International Society for Sandplay Therapy. Prior to the aforementioned events, I had been exposed to sandplay therapy for the first time by another instructor, Dr. Alice Wagstaff, who taught client-centered therapy at the time. Again, I was inexplicably attracted to this therapeutic technique. Dr. Wiersma and Dr. Wagstaff are also both members of the MSTG. In retrospect, my contacts with Dr. Wiersma, Ms. Weller, and Dr. Wagstaff paved the way for my enthusiastic participation in the unique and intriguing world of sandplay. I believe that my encounters with these people were not coincidental. Rather, they were synchronistic events, or what the Taiwanese people would call *u-ian-hun*.

For the first half of my life, I was raised in East Asia, primarily in Taiwan, or Formosa, which means "beautiful island." Growing up in a little town on the island, I was exposed to nature and isolated from the Western, materialistic way of living. I was taught by the elders in town that everything in nature has a spirit. I also played with other children in natural settings near sand, water, and trees. In addition to the emphasis on the importance of my familial relationships (with my nuclear family and with my extended family), there was also a focus on the relationship between people and nature as well. I learned through my ears as well as my eyes and my hands. In Eastern culture and due to the era in which I grew up,

I, as a female, was taught to just "be" rather than to be verbal. Silence was, indeed, golden.

When I turned 16, I had to choose whether I wanted to focus on science or on literature and arts because as a senior in high school, I had to concentrate on one or the other in order to prepare for the entrance exams to either the college of science or the college of literature. At that time in Taiwan, there was no such thing as a liberal arts college. A person had to study either science or literature and arts. Students with exemplary grades were urged to major in the sciences, which is what I chose, although I felt very ambivalent about doing so. One entrance exam would determine which college I would enter and to which department I would be assigned and choices were somewhat limited. I do not believe that it was by chance that I was assigned to the psychology department at the National Taiwan University, which is the most prestigious university in Taiwan. The Department of Psychology was part of the College of the Sciences rather than the College of the Liberal Arts. From that time on, the art and the science of psychology have become a part of my life and my journey.

There was a heavy emphasis on experimental psychology, statistics, and so forth in the Department of Psychology at the National Taiwan University when I attended the program. Even though I was able to obtain good grades in those classes, I felt as if there were something missing from my education. When I graduated, I took a job as a clinical psychologist at the Taipei Children's Mental Health Center. At the time, I thought it was coincidence that I had this job as I did not have any other choice; in retrospect, I think it was another synchronistic event. After working there for two years, I came to the United States to further my education. I obtained my master's degree in psychology in one year. Then, I began to work as a psychologist primarily in the area of assessment, also called evaluation. One of the biggest challenges in conducting psychological assessments was trying to integrate all the psychometric materials in a holistic manner. The question was often this: These are the test results; how do the results relate to one particular individual? The integration of the art and the science of psychology became my quest.

This study provides me with a great challenge because I have to assume dual roles. I have to be both a therapist, which I feel is more related to art, and a researcher, which is more connected with science. In choosing to do this research, I have become the bridge between art and science. Similarly, in becoming a sandplay therapist, I am a bridge between the conscious and the unconscious, the expressed and the hidden, the visible and the invisible, and the external and the internal words of my clients. Since I grew up in Asia in an Eastern, spiritual culture and have lived in the US, thus experiencing the Western, industrialized culture, I believe that I am uniquely qualified to take on the aforementioned dual roles. In this study, I am the researcher as well as the therapist for four of the ten subjects. I would like to emphasize that while

I am the bridge or mediator between research and therapy, my role as therapist takes precedence over my role as researcher. I would never sacrifice the welfare of my clients for the purpose of the research. The clients are my primary concern, and I am indebted to them for their participation in this study.

Now, I would like to briefly describe the sandplay therapy process. Sandplay therapy is an unconventional, creative, primarily nonverbal form of therapy. It utilizes a setting of either one or two sand trays (one filled with wet sand and one filled with dry sand), and the client places miniatures in one of these trays in order to create any type of three-dimensional sand picture. Within the boundaries of therapy's protective environment, the client is free to explore, venture, create, and simply play. In general, the therapist does not physically participate in the creations. Instead, the therapist is an observer and an empathic witness whose active presence facilitates the client's therapeutic process.

When there is a meaningful connection between the client and the therapist, the client is more likely to work out his/her unconscious conflicts through the sandplay process. Symbols play an important role in this process. An example of the conflict between the conscious and the unconscious, and of the importance of symbols, is present in a modern Chinese myth (Christie, 1985, pp. 137–138). This story took place in the province of Yunnan in a village near Horse Year Mountain.

> One year, there was a great drought. All the people of the village were starving because nothing was growing. One day, when Chao and his daughter, the sea girl, went up into the mountains to cut bamboo trees so they could make brooms, they saw a clear and shiny lake. The next day, the sea girl took an axe to the lake because she wanted to make a path so that the water would flow from the lake down to her village. She failed, then sat in despair under a tree, not knowing what to do. A wild goose appeared and informed her that all the girl had to do was find the golden key which would unlock the lake. Before the sea girl could ask the wild goose where she could find the golden key, the wild goose took off.
>
> The girl went into the forest and asked three parrots where she might be able to find the key. They told her, "You have to find the third daughter of the dragon king." Before she could ask where she could find the dragon king's daughter, the three parrots flew off. As the girl was walking home, despondent, a peacock appeared and told her, "Don't despair! You can find the daughter of the dragon king in the canyons of the southern mountains." As the sea girl set off once again on her journey to find the maiden, the peacock flew ahead of her and said, "Wait a minute. Let me tell you that the third daughter of the dragon king enjoys songs that people sing." The sea girl sang folk songs for three days in the

southern mountains, and on the third day, the dragon king's daughter appeared. She admired the sea girl's singing so much, she broke her father's instructions of never entering the human world. The dragon king's daughter asked the sea girl where she was from and why she was singing. The sea girl replied that she needed the key to the lake in order to save the people of her village. The dragon king's daughter answered that she knew where the key was, but it was guarded by an eagle at the dragon king's treasury, and the eagle would kill anyone who went near the treasure. The dragon king's daughter added that she would take the sea girl to the treasury to see what they could do.

The two girls went to the treasury, and as they sang, the eagle woke up, spread his wings, and went to see who was singing. At this moment, the sea girl slipped past him and went into the treasury, which was filled with gold, silver, and jewelry. After resisting her impulse to check out the treasures, the sea girl searched for the key. She accidentally knocked over the box in which the key was hidden. As soon as she found the key, she hurried back to the dragon king's daughter to tell her the good news. The two girls went back to the lake near the sea girl's village. As the sea girl unlocked the lake with the golden key, the water immediately gushed out of the lake. If the dragon king's daughter had not told the sea girl to turn off the flow, the whole town would have been destroyed by the flood. The sea girl used straw screens to stem the threatening flood, then the straw turned into stones. When the dragon king discovered what his daughter had done, he banished her from his kingdom. The dragon king's daughter decided to live with the sea girl, and the two of them sang folk songs together. The women of the village honored the two girls with communal songs on the twenty-second day of the seventh month.

As I was reading this story, I drew an analogy between this myth and how, when we are not in touch with our unconscious lives, a great drought occurs in our conscious lives. This is a story rich with symbols (the birds, the eagle, etc.), but for now, I want to focus on the main story and how it reflects the sandplay process. As a people, we need to find the golden key that will unlock the mystery of our unconscious lives in order to achieve a balance and integration between our unconscious and conscious lives. It is not an easy task to find the key. Additionally, when we do find the key, we may be flooded with unconscious material. It is extremely important to know how to properly transfer the unconscious into the conscious in order for that information to be useful to our conscious lives. In the context of therapy, the better the therapist understands the symbolic meaning of the client's three-dimensional sandplay world, the better their alliance will be, and the easier it is for the client to work out his/her conflicts. Interpretations are not usually done during the session. A review session may be held after the completion of the process at a time determined by the client and the therapist. During this review, the therapist interprets and discusses all of the sand pictures with the client.

In concluding this introduction, I would like to share a dream that I had a few years back. This dream occurred around the time I decided to further my studies and to be a therapist instead of being just an evaluator. In my dream, I was standing on the shore, and I saw a pond filled with sand in a swamp area. Three figures covered with sand rose out of the pond and held out their hands, crying, "Help! Help!" Standing at the shore, I felt compassion for the misery they were experiencing, and I quickly pulled them out of this chaos and brought them to a safe place. At the time of this dream, I did not consciously know that I was on my way to becoming a sandplay therapist.

Chapter 2

Literature review

History of sandplay therapy

Jung had to follow a painful path in order to confront his unconscious (Jung, 1961). After he parted from Freud in 1912, Jung said, "a period of inner uncertainty began for me. It would be no exaggeration to call it a state of disorientation. I felt totally suspended in mid-air, for I had not yet found my own footing" (p. 170). In the midst of his despair, he consciously decided to submit himself to "the impulse of the unconscious" (p. 178). As he was guided by his unconscious, he reluctantly yielded to its command that he build little houses, castles, a village, as well as a church and an altar with the stones he found on the shores of Lake Zurich. This building game became a ritual for him and led to his eventual transformation. In addition to his building, Jung also engaged in active imagination, dream analysis, painting, and stone sculpturing as means of confronting his unconscious. In the end, Jung (1961) concluded:

> The years when I was pursuing my inner images were the most important in my life . . . in them everything essential was decided. It all began then; the later details are only supplements and clarifications of the material that burst forth from the unconscious, and at first swamped me. It was the *primer material* for a lifetime's work. (p. 199)

For Dora Maria Kalff, 1904–1990, the founder of the International Society for Sandplay Therapy, the key to opening the unconscious was sandplay therapy. After spending one year studying at the Lowenfeld's Institute of Child Psychology in London and upon being encouraged by Jung, Kalff synthesized the Lowenfeld approach with a symbolic and archetypal orientation, and she founded *Sandspiel* or *sandplay* (Friedman and Mitchell, 1991). These authors stated:

> Kalff viewed the sandplay process as a natural therapeutic modality that facilitated the expression of the archetypal, symbolic, and intrapersonal

world, as well as everyday alter reality. She believed that the expression of this reality, within a free and protective space created by the therapist, promoted images of wholeness, offering the opportunity for the manifestation of self. Kalff maintained that the manifestation of the self in the tray is necessary, for it serves as a base for the development and strengthening of the ego. When the ego-self connection has been established, the person functions in a more balanced and congruent manner. Through Kalff's many years of observing the process, she realized that the manifestation of the self could be activated by using sandplay with adults as well as with children in an ongoing therapeutic process. (p. 20)

Kalff herself stated (Kalff, 1991):

> The client is given the possibility, by means of figures and by the arrangement of the sand within the area bounded by the sand tray, to set up a world corresponding to his or her inner state. In this manner, through free, creative play, unconscious processes are made visible in a three-dimensional form and in a pictorial world that is comparable to the dream experience. Through a series of images that take shape in this way, the process of individuation, as described by C. G. Jung, is stimulated and brought to fruition. (p. 9)

Kalff's many successful therapeutic examples were illustrated in her book, *Sandplay: A psychotherapeutic approach to the psyche* (Kalff, 1980). What stood out the most about her was her patience, her empathy, her immediate presence, and her wisdom—all of which occurred while she was treating her clients.

In addition to sandplay, she also suggested that when working with children, games and creative activities such as using modeling clay and painting should be employed. She noted that "such games can make an important contribution to the enactment and realization of that which comes to light in the sand images themselves and also, conversely, can further encourage the continuation of the internal sandplay process" (Kalff, 1991, p. 14). Making use of Eric Neumann's "the stages in the child's ego-development" (Neumann, 1990), Kalff remarked that her experience with children and sandplay was similar in that in the beginning of sandplay therapy, themes of the plant and animal worlds would emerge. She called this the animal-vegetative state. She added that the next stage is the fighting stage, which occurs in puberty. She termed the last stage of development as the adaptation to the collective. This is when one resolves conflicts and becomes a member of the collective (Kalff, 1980, pp. 32–33).

Two other well-known therapists who used sandplay or other innovative therapeutic techniques were Agnes "Nessie" Bayley and Ruth Daugherty of England. In March of 1992, they came to Minnesota to conduct advanced training in attachment therapy. In this training, Bayley taught participants about a carefully planned exercise in sensory awareness, which evoked feelings that had been repressed. This exercise would help a therapist to establish bonds with and attachments to his/her clients. Ruth Daugherty, a colleague of Bayley's, having used touch therapy in her work as a social worker with delinquent children, taught participants in the session touch therapy. Daugherty believed that many of these children were deprived of good touch when they were young and that a therapist's appropriate use of good touch would help build a connection between the therapist and the client, promoting therapeutic change.

Katherine Bradway of San Francisco was also influential in the sandplay therapy movement. In 1987, she addressed the International Congress of Analytical Psychology at Einsiedeln, Switzerland with a speech entitled, "What makes it work?" (Bradway, 1987). She illustrated this wonderful therapeutic process by describing a client of hers who came into her office and worked in the sand tray with repetitive and rhythmic movements, such as patting and smoothing an oval island which he had made. Bradway indicated that the event proved to be very healing for the client as well as for her, even though there were no verbal exchanges, no amplifications, and no interpretation.

In April of 1993, Bradway conducted a workshop in Minneapolis. She presented a client of hers with whom sandplay therapy was used in order to help prepare her (the client) to die. This case was published in the *Journal of Sandplay Therapy* (Bradway, 1992). This client, terminally ill with cancer, visited Bradway twenty times in twenty-one months and created fourteen sand trays. Towards the end of the therapy, the client appeared ready to die, and, in fact, died very peacefully. Bradway's tenacity with her clients, combined with her ability to understand what they had experienced, appeared to have caused the therapeutic changes in this particular client.

At the aforementioned workshop, Bradway also described the effects of transference and countertransference in sandplay therapy. She published an article on this topic in the *Journal of Sandplay Therapy* (Bradway, 1991). She illustrated the importance of the transference and countertransference that occurred with her clients' sand pictures and designated the intersection of the two co-transference. She noted:

> A few years ago I found that I was avoiding the use of the term countertransference. I preferred the term co-transference which indicates a feeling with, rather than a feeling against. Currently, I tend to use the term co-transference to designate the therapeutic feeling relationship. These inter-feelings seem to take place more simultaneously than the composite term transference/countertransference suggests. These feelings are, I believe, necessarily determined by both earlier and current happenings. They are, of course, both positive and negative, conscious and

unconscious. And it is not just the person coming for therapy who projects; the therapist does also. Both may find hooks in the other on which to project, or hang, the unused parts of themselves, or repressed parts, or personal images from the past, or archetypal images. And both respond to these projections. One can't help but be affected by the projections of significant others. Moreover, both projections and responses are often entirely at an unconscious level. The therapeutic relationship is a mix; a complex mix; a valuable mix. It is to this mix that I am referring when I use the term co-transference. (Bradway, 1991, p. 29)

At the "Sand, Psyche, and Symbol" conference which was held in San Rafael, California, in 1992, the three prominent therapists who delivered the main speeches were Martin Kalff, son of Dora Kalff; Estelle Weinrib, a practicing therapist in New York; and Hayao Kawai, a Jungian sandplay therapist who practices in Japan. Martin Kalff's talk, entitled "The development of love," included reference to the sandplay processes of two girls and to Buddhist creation myths. His warmth, gentleness, and empathy were on display during his presentation. In an article he wrote for the *Journal of Sandplay Therapy* (Kalff, M., 1993), Kalff brought up an important message about the interpretation of sandplay. He said:

Interpretative skills certainly can help the therapist/counselor enhance and clarify an understanding of the sandplay work in process. This understanding may be used indirectly in the interactions with the client. The capacity to form ideas about the contents of the process within the therapeutic situation, however, is secondary only to the more important capacity of understanding and participating in the process of the client on a preverbal level. The formation of ideas is only a minor element in the general task of forming a relationship with the client that is based on the ideas of the "free and protective space." Too many concepts and fixed ideas about the symbolic process and the expectations based on them create the risk of hampering the capacity of the therapist to remain nonjudgmental and open. On the other hand, it is also true that a deepened capacity of interpreting sandplay brings about respect for the way the individuation process can unfold. Thus it protects one from misjudgment, premature and wrong interventions, and tends to strengthen the trust in the inner healing capacity within the client.

Some clients may feel a need to review the slides of the process with the therapist after concluding their work. It in on this level of the interaction that an interpretation of the scenes on a verbal level can be attempted with the active participation of the client and can prove very rewarding. (Kalff, M., 1993, p. 20)

Estelle Weinrib, the author of a book called *Images of the Self: The sandplay therapy process* (Weinrib, 1983), gave a speech on "What is a sandplay process?" She argued that a successful sandplay process would involve a shift in consciousness, contact with archetypal energy, and a return to an integrated state. She believed that, throughout life, one must return again and again and be reminded of the well-being of the Self. In addition, even though Weinrib attended the conference, her speech was presented in tape form due to her ill health. When she went to the podium, there was thunderous applause, reflecting the enormous appreciation from every participant for her speech and for her lifetime of work as a sandplay therapist. *Images of the Self: The sandplay therapy process* contains many valuable fundamental materials for sandplay therapy, and it is a must-read for all beginning sandplay therapists. The following three paragraphs are a summary of what Weinrib had to say about the important function of the sandplay approach and what benefits it offered.

Sandplay provides direct access to the personal inner world. It creates a creative play world of childhood as well as a fairly safe entry into the deeper archetypal realm, as it gives shapes to and frees the archetypal language of images. It is a means of recovering the specifically feminine dimension of the psyche. It helps repair damage done to the mother-image that would otherwise be detrimental to the integration of the whole personality. Sandplay does this by reconstituting the mother–child unit cohesively, which activates the Self. This is a precursor to the formation of a healthy ego.

In addition, sandplay therapy initiates the instinctual self-healing of the psyche. A "relativization of the ego" can be produced, as well as a more naturally balanced relationship between the ego and the Self. This awakening is a constant theme in sandplay, which also helps inarticulate patients to break through their inner isolation. When they place the miniatures in the tray, they are communicating through the sand pictures. For a therapist who does not have a particularly well-honed intuition or sense of empathy, sand pictures are ideal as they are tangible expressions of the patient's inner world.

Sandplay is also a way to rechannel and/or transform blocked energy. It is a means of self-discovery and awakens a client's creativity without much input from the therapist. It is a rite of passage. At the minimum, sandplay offers an opportunity to explore one's creative and nonrational side, rather than overemphasize the ego-oriented intellect.

As an Asian person, I was most impressed by Hayao Kawai's talk entitled "Sandplay and relation" at this convention. Kawai is known as the founder of the sandplay (*hakoniwa*) therapy in Japan. The minute he reached the podium, Kawai immediately captured everyone's attention by joking about the differences between Western and Eastern cultures concerning how one responds to praise. Later, he skillfully used Japanese stories to illustrate how therapists could enable individuals to recover their lost relationships with others. In his speech, Kawai also mentioned how sandplay therapy had been an effective tool for therapists in Japan to treat children with school phobia. He was very inspiring because of his pioneering spirit and because of his capacity to compare, contrast, and integrate Japanese and Western fairytales (see Kawai, 1988). In Japan, the sandplay therapy is widely used because of Kawai's and several other colleagues' pioneering efforts.

Ruth Ammann, an experienced therapist and author, also expressed her views on sandplay therapy. Ammann (1991) offered the following observation:

> A sand picture can also be seen as the garden of one's soul where the inner and the outer come together. Here, in protected space, a person can learn to watch and recognize the reciprocal action between the inner and the outer world. (p. 12)

Ammann also observed that playing with dry sand is helpful for children to work out childhood issues. Some people may be filled with a deep sadness as they touch the sand because of their desire to be touched lovingly by others. She made one more cogent point:

> When mixed with water, the sand gets ever darker and begins to take on the quality of earth. The sand becomes firm and may be formed or shaped. Now we can create landscapes or three-dimensional structures of all kinds . . . But the sand pictures or sculptures do not remain. They do not become firmer and more nearly permanent as they dry, as with, for example a figure made of clay. In a short time the sand sculpture falls apart and disintegrates. (p. 23)

She added that it was exactly due to this nature that sand pictures are "images of the soul made visible" (p. 23).

Another area of concern is the development aspects of the sandplay. In a review of the available literature, there were two articles that addressed the developmental stages of children during their sandplay process (Bradway, 1990; Stewart, 1990). Based on Neumann, Ericksen, and Piaget's models, Stewart (1990, p. 49) proposed a hypothesis that contains four stages of development in the first twelve years of a child's life:

> Infancy (Inf II): 7–10 to 12–24 months
> Early Childhood I (EC I): 1–2 to 3–4 years
> Early Childhood II (EC II): 3–4 to 6–7 years
> Middle Childhood (MC): 6–7 to 11–12 years.

Some of Stewart's examples in sandplay for Stage 1 were: the behavior of burying and digging up, covering and uncovering, hiding and finding in the sand. The sand text that Stewart presented for the Stage 2 development had to do with order and disorder in the context of various objects which were placed in the sand. For Stage 3, his illustrations demonstrated that there were central-person patterns in the sand text. The Stage 4 sand pictures that

Stewart's clients had created reflected the organization of the developmental stages and objectified the analytic process.

In a similar manner, Bradway (1990) noted that it was helpful for a therapist to relate the child's sand worlds to the stages of ego development propounded by Neumann (1990, p. 139) as five stages and by Doris Kalff as three stages. Neumann's five stages were:

The phallic-chthonian stage of the ego

   a) vegetative
   b) animal

The magic-phallic stage of the ego
The magic-warlike stage of the ego
The solar-warlike stage of the ego
The solar-rational stage of the ego.

Kalff's three stages were: animal-vegetative, fighting, and adaptation to the collective. While it is not necessary to communicate the observations of stages to the child, Bradway (1990) made a point that "an appreciation of what the sand worlds are depicting and an empathy for the struggles and the achievements which the child encounters are conducive to providing *temenos* (Kalff's 'free and sheltered space') within which development will occur" (p. 100).

Addressing the developmental stages of sandplay process, Weinrib (1983) noted that the pictures created in the first phase of the sandplay process usually represented realistic themes and may indicate problems and their possible resolutions. According to Weinrib, the pictures in the second phase often indicated rapid penetration into deeper levels of the personality, into the shadow (personal unconscious). She believed that as the process moved on, one began to see varying degrees of resolutions of the client's problems and complexes. As a result, more energy would be released from the client, which would enable the sandplayer to venture deeper into the psyche to the point where the Self or totality can be touched. Following the self-realization in sandplay, the experience of the transpersonal may be reiterated and reinforced in a conscious way. Weinrib noted it was at this point that the sandplayer was likely to experience a sense of awe and surprise at the richness within him/her. One can usually see the emergence of the rebirth of the ego in the sand pictures at this point. The subsequent pictures then take on a more creative nature, a more organized fashion.

Finally, as mentioned earlier, Dora Kalff founded the International Society for Sandplay Therapy in 1985. This organization is still young and has a limited number of members. Guidelines for training to become a sandplay therapist have been established. The requirements to become a certified sandplay therapist are very stringent. Sandplay therapy can be a powerful tool which may be easily misused; therefore, it needs to be strictly regulated. Both

Dora Kalff (1980, p. 8) and Estelle Weinrib (1983, p. xiv) had the following caution printed in the beginning of their books. The warning stated:

> In the hands of a properly prepared therapist, sandplay is a powerful, invaluable modality. The operative word is "powerful". To the extent that any method can heal, so can it do harm.
>
> Therefore, I urgently advise that even a psychotherapist highly experienced in other methodologies, who contemplates practicing sandplay, should have had a deep personal experience doing a sandplay process as a patient with a qualified sandplay therapist and an extended period of careful supervision—anything less would be irresponsible.

Sandplay therapy outcome research

Case study research

Case study research has been a primary form of investigation concerning the outcome of the sandplay process. In her book, *Sandplay: A psychotherapeutic approach to the psyche*, Dora Kalff (1980) carefully documented the progress of nine cases: seven children, a young woman, and a young man. The usefulness of the sandplay therapy was demonstrated by the following: a 9-year-old boy who overcame an anxiety neurosis; the cure of a 12-year-old boy's learning inhibition; a 12-year-old girl's successful separation from an overpowering mother-fixation; a 16-year-old boy who worked on his loss of instinct due to his identification with an extroverted mother; a 5½-year-old boy's triumph over a speech block; a young, adopted girl who overcame her inability to read; a 23-year-old woman's restoration of a weak ego; and a 25-year-old man who defeated his embarrassment at and annoyance of blushing easily.

In her book *Images of the Self*, Estelle Weinrib (1983) carefully presented a case study which she labeled as a relatively short process. She concluded that significant growth and real change in this young man had occurred in the following areas:

- The father complex was largely resolved, as was the identification with the intellect.
- There was a period of intense confusion with the emergence of the sensation/reality function and the previously repressed feeling.
- The incipient paranoid delusional system and the dangerous inflation was arrested, as was the crippling obsessive compulsivity.
- Differentiation of masculine and feminine functioning occurred.
- As his own feeling evolved, he withdrew the anima projection from his woman friend and found that he could love her. But she was apparently

unable to adjust to the loss of control of the relationship, and so it foundered.
- He changed his lifestyle and left his therapy with feeling of buoyancy and optimism, mixed with sadness and some anxiety. (pp. 156–157)

Other authors and therapists who have written about the outcome of their sandplay therapy processes with children and adults include John Allan (1988), Joel Ryce-Menuhin (1988), Kaspar Kiepenheuer (1990), and Ruth Ammann (1991). Allan, through the sandplay process, helped a second-grade boy reduce his impulsive and aggressive behavior. Ryce-Menuhin helped a 3½-year-old adopted child achieve a more healthy adjustment to being adopted. Kiepenheuer treated a young woman and a young man overcome by depression. Ammann's case reports included a 40-year-old woman who triumphed over severe depression and another 40-year-old woman who made a successful process of feminine transformation. In addition, Ammann also documented the process of a 7-year-old girl who exhibited a disturbance in her primal relationship with her mother and disturbances in her social behavior. Ammann commented that after thirty-three hours of therapy, this girl was able to develop a healthy ego and a stronger personality.

In an effort to obtain more literature concerning the efficacy of sandplay therapy, a literature search was performed. Unfortunately, data were rather limited. Most outcome studies were based on case reports. Successful case presentations were also presented by other authors in various journal articles: Allan and Berry (1987), Vinturella and James (1987), Carey (1990), Miller and Boe (1990), and Zappacosta (1992). Zappacosta (1992), in particular, stressed the importance of the divine energies in play. Zappacosta believed that the recovery of these energies was the way to strengthen and synthesize the entire personality.

Objective study

The majority of the objective studies for sandplay used sandplay results as a projective technique. While using sandplay as a projective test was not a popular trend at this time (Mitchell and Friedman, 1992), at least three studies (Domenico and Schubach, 1987; Caproni and Martin, 1989; Segal, 1990) attempted to gain knowledge in this realm. Even though it is likely that a sand tray represents something which is projected from the unconscious, it must be used with caution as a diagnostic tool. At the same time, however, a therapist must value the possible indicative information that is conveyed in the sand tray; thus, the therapist is more likely to be an empathic witness to the process, rather than a passive observer.

No objective outcome study of the sandplay process was found in the literature read for this study. The only objective study of the sandplay process known to the author included a project which was conducted by the

Minnesota Sandplay Therapy Group at the same site as this study, under the direction of Dr. Lawrence Greenberg, a child psychiatrist at the University of Minnesota. In that study, Dr. Greenberg employed the Kendall Self-Rating Scale and the Self-Perception Profile for Children as outcome indicators. Communication with him revealed that the results from his study indicated a definite, but nonsignificant trend towards improvement in six of the eight subjects in the experimental group. There was no such indication in any of the subjects in the control group.

Psychotherapy outcome research

This section will briefly explain the problems and limitations with regard to psychotherapy outcome research. Due to the complexity of this issue and to the limitations of this study, this review will focus on the issues brought up by Strupp (1973), who substantially contributed to the field of psychotherapy outcome. His investigations appeared to be quite thorough. He examined a number of variables associated with the therapist's personality and attributes, the therapeutic techniques, and the interactional variables between the therapist and the client. Furthermore, he pointed out that increasing efforts were being made in regard to studying the client's life situations and other environmental factors. Strupp also noted that in psychotherapy, the dual roles of clinician and researcher were difficult to reconcile. The clinician has been viewed as the artist, while the researcher is deemed a scientist, and their respective approaches have been regarded as antithetical and mutually exclusive. While greater collaboration between the dual roles is desirable and has started to occur, the marriage between the two has been an uneasy one. Strupp (1973) remarked:

> As researchers we seem to lack methods for making greater inroads on the phenomena with which psychotherapy deals—the broad spectrum of human experience. For instance, how do we assess and measure such qualities in the therapist as respect for the patient's struggle toward self-realization and self-direction, capacity for empathy, warmth, acceptance of the human-ness of another person, depth of one's *Weltanschauung* and life experience, emotional maturity, ability to serve as a model of reality, and so forth—all of which undoubtedly play an important role in determining the extent to which the therapist can participate in and collaborate with the patient's striving for realizing his human potentialities? By contrast, the quantitative and comparative analyses of technique, formidable as they are, appear like child's play. (pp. 753–754)

Strupp went on to state that the techniques for measuring significant personality attributes are in their infancy and that contributions from researchers to psychotherapeutic theory and practice have been relatively scarce. He further challenged clinicians and researchers to take on the task, if it is not an impossible task, to integrate the art and the science of psychotherapy. Another quote from Strupp (1973) concludes this chapter:

> The task poses a great challenge to our imagination as researchers. We must show greater penetration in forging our research tools and refuse to purchase precision at the expense of shallowness of concepts. If we agree to the proposition that psychotherapy's future is that of a scientific discipline, we have no choice but to undertake the laborious and painful drudgery of checking the empirical value of brilliant clinical insights glimpsed by intrepid pioneers and to sharpen our research instruments that they may become adequate to deal with the phenomena in our domain. It is just barely possible that a few crumbs of insight left over by the giants may be the reward of the patient researcher, not to mention the gratification of demolishing along the way some hypotheses that contemporaneously enjoy the status of a creed. (p. 754)

Chapter 3
Method

Location of study

The selected site of this study was a small, parochial school located in the inner city of Minneapolis. A similar study was conducted during the 1991–1992 school year, but it did not include such extensive pre-therapy and post-therapy measures. During that previous study, an unfortunate event took place (a subject of the study was expelled from school before therapy could be completed). Consequently, the Minnesota Sandplay Therapy Group (MSTG) prepared a Mission Statement for the current study, to be signed by both the MSTG and the school principal. This effort was made in order to protect the therapeutic experience of every subject.

Subjects

Initially, more than ten subjects were chosen by the school social worker based on their need for therapy. This social worker had close contact with every child in this school and knew which children needed mental help the most. The final decision of the ten subjects was made based on the interaction between the research team and the social worker, and on the availability of the parents to sign a consent form for the study. In the final determination of which students would receive therapy, the children's needs took precedence over the other factors.

In order to aid the therapy of each child, a list of referral notes was provided by the social worker to the research team, which consisted of four therapists, a supervisor, a project director, and Dr. Lawrence Greenberg, who collected the results of the Kendall Self-Rating Scale and the Self-Perception Profile for Children. In order to protect the confidentiality of the children, the pertinent information about these subjects is summarized in a global manner. First of all, the majority of the children were non-white, and all but one were female. Three out of the ten students were in the upper elementary school grades, and three were in the lower elementary school grades. The rest of the subjects were in the intermediate elementary school grades. More than half of the children lived in single-parent households. Child Protection has been involved with at least three of the children in the past. Some of the problems listed for the children include: witnessing violence; sexual abuse; alcohol and drug use in the family. One child witnessed the violent murder of a cousin by her stepfather, who was then placed in jail. One child's father (in jail at this time) has repeatedly attempted to kill the child and the mother. On the birthday of one of the children, her brother tried to kill himself. Yet another child was brutally sexually abused by a neighbor years ago. Child Protection and the police failed to convict or remove the perpetrator, who continued to live next door to this child. Another child was suspected to be the victim of incest. Another child had scoliosis and had to wear a brace, as well as experiencing hearing loss and visual problems. One subject was suspected to be nearly psychotic.

Procedure

Chosen pre- and post-therapy test instruments were:

1 Children Depression Inventory (CDI) (Kovacs, 1979). The CDI is a twenty-seven item self-report measure of a child's depression. This test was individually administered and read to the younger subjects by the evaluator.
2 Rorschach (Exner Method) (Exner, 1986; Exner and Weiner, 1986).
3 Teacher's Report Form (TRF) (Achenbach, 1991). The form was chosen over the parent's form because the social worker at this school did not think that the parents would cooperate in filling out the form.
4 House-Tree-Person (H-T-P) drawings.

The CDI, the Rorschach, and the H-T-P drawings were given to the children within one to two weeks prior to and post-therapy. All pre-therapy tests were administered by the author. She administered all of the post-therapy tests to the subjects who did not have her as their therapist. Another evaluator, a child psychologist, administered the post-therapy tests to the subjects for whom the author was the therapist. The TRF were filled out by the homeroom teacher within the same time frame. All of the subjects were given twenty therapy sessions, which included sandplay therapy as one of the available techniques. One subject chose to terminate therapy after eighteen sessions. The rest of the subjects completed all twenty sessions. For the purpose of this study, the subjects will be referred to by numbers one to ten. All therapists were asked to write a brief summary of the changes, both positive and negative, which they saw in the children during the twenty sessions.

Therapy

The therapy was conducted in a large room in the basement of the school. In this room, there was an area which was used for the sandplay process. In this area, there were two standing sand trays, one containing wet sand and the other containing dry sand. There was one large cabinet, two small cabinets, and one bookcase. The cabinets and the bookcase all contained and displayed miniatures. The miniatures were provided by the MSTG and included: items of nature, such as rocks, stones, shells, and trees of various types; animals, including wild, domestic, prehistoric, and fantasy animals; human beings, such as people of different races, families, babies, fantasy figures, people with different occupations; religious items; transportation and buildings; furniture and food items; other miscellaneous items.

A water container was also in the room, providing the children with the opportunity to make the sand wetter if they wished. Another corner of the playroom was the art area. In this corner, there was an easel, paint, fingerpaint, crayons and markers, stickers, clay, and flour-based modeling compound. Another area of the playroom was carpeted and equipped with various games and toys. For each therapy session, the children could choose to do whatever they wanted. During the initial session, the school social worker, who knew the child well, explained the purpose of the therapy before introducing the child to the therapist. Then, the child was left alone with the therapist. The therapist explicitly explained to the child how long the session would be (forty minutes), how many sessions there would be (twenty), and about confidentiality. The child was instructed that s/he could choose to participate in any activity which s/he preferred. Some of the choices included: talking, playing a game, playing with toys, painting, drawing, sculpting, and sandplay. In regards to sandplay, the child was informed that s/he could put any miniature into either of the trays in any way s/he wished. S/he could also add water to the wet tray if s/he wanted the sand to be wetter. The therapist also allowed the child to know that s/he would receive a five-minute warning before the end of the session so s/he could complete the picture s/he was creating. All sand pictures and art products were photographed after each session, and during the final session, each child was given a complete set of pictures to keep. In addition, a definite day and time for therapy was set. Every therapist and her child held a party during the last session, which also included going over all the sand pictures.

Therapists

In addition to the author, three other therapists were chosen by the Minnesota Sandplay Therapy Group as interns. All of the therapists worked in the mental health field and have completed their own sandplay therapy processes. All of the therapists were beginning sandplay therapists, working toward their certification. With the exception of the author, who is Asian, the rest of the therapists were Caucasian. All of the therapists were female. The author was the therapist of four subjects whereas the other three therapists had two subjects each. Group supervision was provided on a regular basis by Barbara Weller, a certified member of the International Society for Sandplay Therapy.

Other considerations

Since most of the subjects came from very unstable backgrounds, special steps were taken in order to prevent the traumatic effects of abandonment. For example, a child was given something to keep as a transitional object when the therapist went away on a vacation or on holidays. Calendars were available for each child so that s/he could keep track of sessions and the number of remaining sessions. A globe was used to illustrate to a child where the therapist was when she went on vacation. Since most of the children formed strong attachments to their therapists, special care was taken by each therapist to minimize possible detrimental effects of the therapist's absence.

In spite of these meticulous preparations, special unavoidable events took place. For one thing, the author had to go back to Taiwan for her brother's funeral in November, 1992, which was when the subjects were first seen. The most devastating event, however, occurred from the middle until the end of this study. During the month of December, there was a rumor that the school might be closing. Attempts were made by the therapists to write to the appropriate authorities to prevent the closing of the school. These attempts failed, and the final decision to close the school was announced in February of 1993.

These children loved their school and often felt at a loss when the school was not in session. It would not be an exaggeration to say that the school was equally as important as, if not more important than, the families to the children. The closing of the school would take place at the end of the school year. This was crushing news not only for the students, but also for the children who were in this study, the school staff, and the therapists. The effect the closing of the school had on this study will be explained in the discussion section.

Scoring of the tests

All of the tests which the author had administered were scored by her. All of the post-therapy tests administered by another psychologist to the author's subjects were scored by that psychologist and the author together. An experienced child psychologist, Jana Hutchinson, PhD, Licensed Psychologist, did a blind interpretation of the ten sets of Rorschach protocols, plus Structural Summaries. She was instructed to do a global evaluation, contrasting and comparing each pair of protocols for each subject. Only minimal information was provided about the subjects, such as grade level, gender, and racial background. The evaluator did not know which of the protocols were the pre and post for each subject. Another experienced child psychologist, Regina Driscoll, PhD, Licensed Psychologist, did a blind interpretation of the H-T-P drawings. Again, she compared and contrasted the sets of pre- and post-therapy drawings of each subject; she also gave a global rating for each subject. In this case, she did not know the age, gender, or racial background of the subjects. She also did not know which set had the pre-therapy drawings and which had the post-therapy drawings.

Chapter 4
Results and discussion

The findings will be presented in the following order: the results and discussion of the Children Depression Inventory; the results and discussion of the Rorschach, based on Structural Summaries and blind interpretations; the results and discussion of the Teacher's Report Form; the results and discussion of the House-Tree-Person drawings blind interpretations and therapists' reports. In addition, the results of the Rorschach Structural Summaries will be subdivided into the following categories: cognition; affect; self-perception; interpersonal perception and relations; capacity for self-control and stress tolerance. The variables chosen for each category will be presented in the tables provided for each result.

Children Depression Inventory

The CDI is a twenty-seven item, self-report measure of children's depression. The test is derived from the Beck Depression Inventory for Adults. Each statement in each item is scored from zero to two, with two as the choice for the most severe depressive symptoms. Even though there are no well-established cutoff scores to classify the level of the severity of depression in the CDI as there are in the inventory for adults, a common cutoff suggested in determining depression for out-patients is twelve. For in-patients, it is fifteen. In Table 4.1, the subject's pre- and post-therapy test scores are presented. In addition, their scores on the suicide item (item 9) are presented as well because this is the most important item at the pre-therapy test level. This item consists of the following sentence:

> I do not think about killing myself (score zero); I think about killing myself, but would not do it (score one); I want to kill myself (score two).

The pre-therapy scores of three subjects (Subjects 3, 7, 9) were above the cutoff score of twelve, which is commonly used for out-patient referrals. Of the three, two of the subjects' post-therapy test scores (Subjects 3, 7) were within the normal range. Clear gains were shown in these two subjects.

Table 4.1 The results of the Children Depression Inventory (CDI)

Subjects	Pre	Post	Suicide item (item 9) Pre	Post
1	1	0	0	0
2	6	7	0	0
3	24	8	1	0
4	2	2	1	0
5	2	3	1	0
6	1	0	1	0
7	13	9	1	1
8	6	0	1	0
9	32	30	2	1
10	2	0	0	0

Since the pre-therapy test scores were within the normal range for the other subjects, they did not have any room for improvement. However, the author would like to note that Subject 8 showed improvement, too. The pre-therapy score was six while the post-therapy score was zero.

Perhaps the biggest improvement shown on this test had to do with the suicidal potential of the subjects. Five of the subjects changed from "I think about killing myself, but would not do it" to "I do not think about killing myself." In addition, one subject changed from "I want to kill myself" to "I think about killing myself, but would not do it." In addition, three of the subjects (Subjects 1, 2, 10) scored zero on this item for both the pre- and post-therapy tests, meaning that they never thought about killing themselves. Only Subject 7 did not show improvement, with pre- and post-therapy test scores of one, meaning the subject consistently thought, "I think about killing myself, but would not do it."

Rorschach

As previously indicated, the first part of the Rorschach results is based on the pre- and post-Structural Summaries and is presented in the following categories: cognition; affect; self-perception; interpersonal perception and relations; capacity for control and tolerance for stress. The author compared norms taken from Exner's Rorschach Workbook (Exner, 1990) with the subjects' scores. Since the norms used were for the subjects' age groups, the maturity factory (the subject's maturity that s/he accrued over the six months of therapy) could be considered negligible.

Cognition

The variables chosen for this category were $X+\%$, $F+\%$, $X-\%$, $Xu\%$, *WSUM 6*, *Schizophrenia Index*, and *Popular Responses*. A brief explanation of the meaning of each variable based on Exner's Comprehensive System follows:

1   $X+\%$ (Conventional Form) concerns perceptual accuracy for the total record. For interpretation, the $X+\%$ provides data related to the use of the form features of the blot in a commonplace, reality-oriented manner.
2   $F+\%$ (Conventional, Pure Form) concerns accuracy among the pure F responses. It was postulated by Beck that when the quality of the form used is good, the subject demonstrates a respect for reality, whereas the frequent use of a poor form indicates a disregard for this element.
3   $X-\%$ (Distorted Form) concerns the proportion of perceptual distortion which has occurred in the record. When a subject's $X-\%$ is greater than 15 percent, there is concern that s/he has difficulty in translating perceptual input appropriately or accurately.
4   $Xu\%$ (Unusual Form) concerns the proportion of answers in which contours have been used appropriately, but unconventionally.
5   *WSUM 6* is based on six Critical Special Scores—Deviant Verbalization, Incongruous Combination, Deviant Response, Fabulized Combination, Inappropriate Logic, and Contamination. The *WSUM 6* is used to identify events in which some difficulties occur in cognitive processing.
6   *Schizophrenia Index* represents the sum of the number of variables which are positive for criterion in a cluster of variables related to problems in thinking and perpetual accuracy.
7   *Popular Responses* relates to the ability to perceive and to respond to the commonplace features of the blot. A low frequency of popular responses in a record often reflects either an inability or an unwillingness on the part of the subject to deliver what would be considered the most possible answer.

In Table 4.2, pre- and post-test results for these variables are presented. An asterisk signifies that the score was two standard deviations below the mean for that age group. Two asterisks indicate that the score was two standard deviations above the mean for that age group.

Clear improvement was demonstrated in four of the subjects (Subjects 3, 4, 6, 8) in their *WSUM 6* results. Furthermore, a substantial gain was shown in three of the subjects (Subjects 1, 4, 6) in their *Schizophrenic Index*, using four as a cutoff score. Four of the subjects (Subjects 4, 5, 6, 9) showed marked gain in their $F+\%$. Two of the subjects (Subjects 1, 4) exhibited positive change in their $X-\%$ as well. In addition, five of the subjects (Subjects 3, 6, 7, 8, 9) improved in their *Popular Responses*. The results of $X+\%$ and $Xu\%$ were not as consistent; some subjects improved while other subjects deteriorated.

Table 4.2 Rorschach results: cognition

Subjects	X+% Pre	X+% Post	F+% Pre	F+% Post	X–% Pre	X–% Post	Xu% Pre	Xu% Post	WSUM6 Pre	WSUM6 Post	SCZI Pre	SCZI Post	P Pre	P Post
1	0.40*	0.60	0.47	0.67	0.32*	0.13	0.28*	0.27	9	2	4	0	8	6
2	0.71	0.59	0.67	0.55	0.00	0.12	0.29*	0.29*	6	0	0	0	6	6
3	0.14*	0.26*	0.00*	0.20*	0.36*	0.37*	0.45*	0.30*	32**	2	5	4	3*	6
4	0.27*	0.43*	0.25*	0.36	0.36*	0.14	0.32*	0.43*	36**	2	4	1	4	2*
5	0.39*	0.58*	0.43*	0.55	0.22*	0.21*	0.39*	0.32*	16	8	2	1	6	6
6	0.22*	0.50*	0.25*	0.47	0.53*	0.25*	0.25	0.25	58**	15	6	2	4*	5
7	0.15*	0.22*	0.50	0.32*	0.69*	0.69*	0.15	0.09	52**	51**	6	5	2*	5
8	0.71	0.56*	1.00	0.50	0.14	0.06	0.14	0.38*	23**	8	3	1	1*	7
9	0.24*	0.29*	0.14*	1.00	0.48*	0.47*	0.28*	0.24	58**	30**	6	5	4*	7
10	0.43*	0.56*	0.44*	0.59	0.12	0.18	0.32*	0.40	7	0	1	1	6	7

* 2 SD below the mean for subject's age group
** 2 SD above the mean for subject's age group

Overall, of the subjects who demonstrated poor reality testing and poor cognition at the pre-therapy level, most of them improved remarkably in these areas.

Affect

The variables chosen for this category were *EB*, *eb*, *FC:CF+C*, *Afr*, and *S*. Following is a brief explanation as to what each variable means:

1. *EB* (Erlebnistypus) represents a relationship between two major variables —human movement and the weighted sum of the chromatic color responses. The directionality of this ratio, such as introversive, extratensive, and ambitent, indicates the preferential response style of the individual. Exner proposed that the directionality of the *EB* is far less stable in children, and the ambitent appears to me much more vulnerable to intra or interpersonal problems.
2. *eb* (Experience Base) represents a relationship which compares all nonhuman movement determinants with the shading and achromatic color determinants. It is known to provide information concerning stimuli demands experienced by the subject.
3. *FC:CF+C* (Form-Color Ratio) provides an index of the extent to which emotional discharges are modulated. It is known that *FC* responses equate more with a positive affective experience which has been controlled and/or directed by cognitive elements, whereas *CF+C* illustrates instances in which the subject has been more prone to give in to affective stimulus.
4. *Afr* (Affective Ratio) provides information concerning the responsiveness of a person to emotional stimulation. Elevations signify a tendency towards overresponsiveness, whereas low scores signify avoidance tendencies.
5. *S* (Space Response) represents the answers which included the use of white space. It is known that elevation in *S* suggests possible negativism and the possible existence of anger which is provoked by intense and/or prolonged periods of dissatisfaction. In an average-length record, the presence of one or two *S* responses is likely to be a positive sign, but if there are more than three *S* responses, oppositionality is more likely to be pervasive as a trait-like feature of the individual's personality. A frequency of four or more *S* responses loads positively in the Suicide Constellation.

In Table 4.3, pre- and post-test results for these variables are presented. One asterisk signifies that the score was two standard deviations below the mean for that age group. Two asterisks indicate that the score was two standard deviations above the mean for that age group.

The results were somewhat more ambiguous than those in the Cognitive

Table 4.3 Rorschach: affect

Subjects	EB Pre	EB Post	eb Pre	eb Post	FC:CF+C Pre	FC:CF+C Post	Afr Pre	Afr Post	S Pre	S Post
1	4:3.0	3:4.5	1:0	3:3	0:3	1:4	0.14*	0.50	2	2
2	3:0.0	1:0.5	5:2	4:2	0:0	1:0	0.40*	0.31*	0	0
3	5:8.5	8:5.0	11:9	5:5	0:8	2:3	0.38*	0.42*	4	5
4	0:2.5	0:1.0	5:5	1:2	3:1	0:1	0.47*	0.56*	5	5
5	8:5.0	4:0.5	4:1	4:0	4:3	1:0	0.64	0.64	0	0
6	1:0.0	0:0.0	1:2	1:0	0:0	0:0	0.45*	0.67	2	0
7	5:4.0	3:7.0	4:2	9:4	4:2	4:5	0.44*	0.45*	1	5
8	5:2.5	5:0.5	6:1	8:4	1:2	1:0	0.40*	0.33*	0	0
9	3:10.5	5:2.0	11:1	15:4	1:10	0:2	0.92**	0.21*	0	1
10	0:0.0	1:0.0	6:0	6:2	0:0	0:0	0.33*	0.41*	3	2

* 2 SD below the mean for subject's age group
** 2 SD above the mean for subject's age group

section. Improvement was shown for two subjects (Subjects 1, 6) in their *Afr* scores. *Afr* is known to be related to interest in emotional stimulation. Two subjects (Subjects 3, 9) appeared to have better *FC:CF+C*, which relates to modulation of affect. The results of all the other variables were mixed and did not reveal any significant trend. Overall, in the realm of affect, only a slight gain was seen in a minority of the subjects. This was not surprising in view of the fact that most of the subjects experienced some emotional setbacks during post-therapy when the school closed.

Self-perception

The variables chosen for this category were *3r+(2)/R, Fr+rF, FD, V, MOR, H:(H)+Hd+(Hd)*. Here is the definition of each variable:

1. *3r+(2)/R* (Egocentricity Index) represents the proportion of reflection and pair responses in the total record and is known to relate to self-centeredness. It is also used as a measure of psychological self-focusing or self-concern. An excess of self-concern or a lack of self-concern can both be potential liabilities. A high score signifies an excess of self-centeredness, whereas a low score signals low self-esteem.
2. *Fr+rF* indicates use of reflection in determining a response; *FD* (Form Dimension Responses) demonstrates use of the impression of depth, distance, or dimension in determining a response; *V* (Vista Responses) shows use of the shady features of the blot to explain the impression of depth or dimensionality and is known to be related to one's self-focusing, self-inspection, and self-awareness.
3. *MOR* (Morbid Content) is known to be a suicide indicator and related to

depression in children. The presence of any morbid content is often significant.

4   $H:(H)+Hd+(Hd)$ represents the sum of pure human responses on the left and the sum of other human contents on the right. This ratio provides information about interest in people. The absence of pure H responses often signifies a marked lack of interest in people. A higher score on the right side of this index suggests that self-perception may be distorted and based on fantasies.

In Table 4.4, pre- and post-test results for these variables are listed. An asterisk signifies that the score was two standard deviations below the mean for that age group.

Subjects 1 and 10 appeared to show improvement in their $3r+(2)/R$, which relates to one's self-centeredness. Subjects 1 and 6 also demonstrated improvement in their MOR, which is commonly seen as a suicide indicator. Subjects 4, 5, and 6 were more able to deal with people on a realistic level rather than on a fantasy level, based on their $H:(H)+Hd+(Hd)$. On the whole, there seemed to be only a slight improvement in the subjects' self-perceptions. It is possible that the school's closing bruised their self-perceptions, impeding any more significant progress.

Interpersonal perception and relations

The variables chosen for this category were *CDI*, *T*, *Food*, *Human content*, *a:p*, *Isolate/R*, *COP*, *AG*, *PER*. The descriptions of each follow:

1   *CDI* (Coping Deficit Index) usually indicates that a subject's ability to cope is impaired if the score is above 4 or 5.

Table 4.4 Rorschach: self-perception

Subjects	3r+(2)/R Pre	Post	Fr+rF Pre	Post	FD Pre	Post	V Pre	Post	MOR Pre	Post	H:(H)+Hd+(Hd) Pre	Post
1	0.24*	0.47	0	1	0	1	0	0	1	0	4:3	4:2
2	0.43*	0.29*	0	0	1	0	0	0	1	1	3:0	1:3
3	0.18*	0.37*	0	0	1	1	0	0	1	1	6:3	5:5
4	0.18*	0.07*	0	0	0	0	0	0	1	0	0:10	1:5
5	0.61	0.68	2	2	1	0	0	0	0	1	3:10	3:4
6	0.41	0.45	0	0	0	0	0	0	3	0	2:9	1:2
7	0.08*	0.02*	0	0	0	1	0	1	3	2	0:1	3:2
8	0.71	0.56	2	1	0	0	0	0	0	2	3:0	3:2
9	0.56	0.53	0	0	1	0	0	1	2	1	2:2	4:2
10	0.28*	0.54	0	0	0	0	0	0	1	0	1:7	2:8

* 2 SD below the mean for subject's age group

2. *T* (Texture Determinant) has to do with the responses when the shading components of the blot area are used to justify or clarify these kinds of associations. It is known to reflect a cautious sensitivity and to be related to a willingness to be open to the environment. Elevation signifies greater needs for closeness, whereas a zero score suggests guardedness or distance in interpersonal contacts. *Food* responses are known to be related to one's dependency needs. *Human content* is related to one's interest in interpersonal interactions.

3. *a:p* represents active or passive coding for all movement responses. It is proposed that elevation in the right-hand side of this ratio signifies a potential to take flight into passive forms of fantasy as a defensive maneuver.

4. *Isolate/R* (Isolation Index) provides information concerning one's views and reactions to the social environment. When the left-side value is greater than one-fourth of the right-side value, a marked tendency towards social isolation is suggested.

5. *COP* (Cooperative Movement) is assigned to any movement response involving two or more objects in which the interaction is clearly passive or cooperative.

6. *AG* (Aggressive Movement) is used for any movement response in which the action is clearly aggressive.

7. *PER* (Personal) is assigned to any response in which the subject refers to personal knowledge or experience as part of the basis for justifying and/or clarifying a response. A high score usually signifies a need to be overly precise in defending one's self-image.

In Table 4.5, pre- and post-test results for these variables are listed.

The *AG* scores of subjects 5, 6, 7, 9, and 10 significantly decreased. An elevated *AG* usually indicates an increased likelihood for aggressive behavior. Conversely, the decrease in these subjects' *AG* scores suggests that these subjects are less likely to engage in acting-out behavior. No consistent trend appeared for most of the other variables in this category. The scores of those other variables were not adequate to produce significant information due to the small sampling size of the subjects and to the complexity of these factors.

Capacity for control and tolerance for stress

The variables used for this category were *D*, *Adj D*, *EA*, *es*, and *CDI*. The variables were defined as:

1. *D* (Unadjusted D Score) provides information concerning the relationship between *EA* and *es*. This relates to stress tolerance and elements of control. If a *D* score exceeds zero, it signifies greater capacity for control

Table 4.5 Rorschach: interpersonal perception and relations

Subjects	CDI Pre	CDI Post	T Pre	T Post	Food Pre	Food Post	Human content Pre	Human content Post	a:p Pre	a:p Post	Isolate/R Pre	Isolate/R Post	COP Pre	COP Post	AG Pre	AG Post	PER Pre	PER Post
1	2	1	0	1	1	0	7	6	3:2	4:2	0.16	0.40	2	2	0	0	0	0
2	3	4	1	1	0	0	3	4	6:2	2:3	0.29	0.12	2	1	0	0	0	0
3	3	2	0	1	0	1	9	10	10:6	9:5	0.55	0.33	1	2	1	2	6	1
4	4	4	3	0	1	0	10	6	4:1	1:0	0.00	0.14	3	0	0	0	3	0
5	0	2	1	0	0	0	13	7	8:4	6:2	0.13	0.11	3	4	2	1	3	1
6	3	4	0	0	0	0	11	3	2:0	1:0	0.06	0.00	1	0	1	0	0	0
7	2	4	0	0	1	1	1	5	7:2	10:2	0.15	0.02	0	0	3	0	0	2
8	3	2	0	0	0	0	3	5	6:5	10:4	0.14	0.13	0	0	0	1	1	0
9	0	3	1	0	0	0	4	6	10:5	16:6	0.16	0.59	4	2	3	1	0	0
10	4	4	0	2	0	0	8	10	3:3	5:2	0.00	0.10	1	0	1	0	1	0

and greater tolerance for stress. On the other hand, subjects with *D* scores in the minus range are vulnerable to becoming overwhelmed by external stimuli and to becoming disorganized.
2   *Adj D* (Adjusted D Score) provides information concerning stress tolerance and available resources.
3   *EA* (Experience Actual) is known to relate to available resources.
4   *es* (Experience Stimulation) relates to current stimulus demands.
5   *CDI* (Coping Deficit Index) was defined earlier.

In Table 4.6, pre- and post-test results for these results are listed. An asterisk signifies that the score was two standard deviations below the mean for the subject's age group.

Mixed results also occurred in these areas. Subjects 3 and 4 appeared to establish greater self-control and tolerance for stress, whereas Subjects 7, 8, and 9 displayed deterioration in these areas. One can only speculate once again that some of the subjects, especially the more vulnerable ones, were overwhelmed by the closing of the school.

The second half of the Rorschach results presented here was based on blind interpretations. As previously indicated, Dr. Hutchinson was the rater for ten sets of Rorschach protocols, including Structural Summaries. She was asked to give simple global ratings and to differentiate between the pre-therapy protocol and the post-therapy protocol for each subject. She was correct on nine out of the ten sets. Her only incorrect prediction was for Subject 2. Dr. Hutchinson's prediction as to the pre- and post-therapy protocols are underlined at the beginning of each record. Her list of descriptive terms for each subject's pre-and post protocols then follows each of her predictions. For clarification, 1A was used to denote Subject 1's pre-therapy

Table 4.6 Rorschach: capacity for control and tolerance for stress

Subjects	D Pre	Post	Adj D Pre	Post	EA Pre	Post	es Pre	Post	CDI Pre	Post
1	+2	+0	+2	+0	7.0	7.5	1	6	2	1
2	−1*	−1*	−1*	−1*	3.0	1.5	7	6	3	4
3	−2*	+1	+0	+2	13.5	13.0	20	10	3	2
4	−2*	+0	−2*	+0	2.5	1.0	10	3	4	4
5	+3	+0	+3	+0	13.0	4.5	5	4	0	2
6	+0	+0	+0	+0	1.0	0.0	3	1	3	4
7	+1	−1*	+1	−1*	9.0	10.0	6	13	2	4
8	+0	−2*	+1	−2*	7.5	5.5	7	12	3	2
9	+0	−4*	+1	−3*	13.5	7.0	12	19	0	3
10	−2*	−2*	−1*	−2*	0.0	1.0	6	8	4	4

* 2 SD below the mean for subject's age group

record, and 1B was the designation for Subject 1's post-therapy record, and so forth.

Furthermore, since Dr. Hutchinson was instructed to provide global and brief assessments for each protocol, one could infer from the results that nine out of ten subjects demonstrated improvement in their personality functioning at the post-therapy level. The fact that improvement was not readily shown in the more discrete variables mentioned earlier is likely a result of the limited number of subjects in the study and the limited time frame for experimentation. If there had been more subjects and enough time for the inner changes depicted by the global assessment to manifest, changes might have been seen in the more discrete variables.

1A. *Pre-therapy protocol*: More rigid; poorer form quality; appears overwhelmed by affect; morbid responses of a heart that's been shot.
1B. *Post-therapy protocol*: Less rigid, greater ability to respond to color and affect; better form quality; Texture response; more complex-integrated responses; better self-concept on Card 1.
2A. *Pre-therapy protocol*: Less rigid; less tension; better form quality.
2B. *Post-therapy protocol*: More rigid; rejection of Card IX; inability to do inquiry on Card IV; H response with minus quality.
3A. *Pre-therapy protocol*: More tension, such as dynamite blowing up, volcano erupting, smoke-thunderstorm.
3B. *Post-therapy protocol*: Still many abstract perceptions, but more happy, positive ones in this protocol; better form quality; not as distressed.
4A. *Pre-therapy protocol*: More reactive, responsive, but percepts are "scary," "has head cut off"; many indicators of distress and neediness.
4B. *Post-therapy protocol*: Well-defended; better reality testing; attempts were made to integrate; D/Adj D equals zero, suggesting subject is not as distressed; WSUM 6 score significantly better.
5A. *Pre-therapy protocol*: Not as rigid or defensive as other protocol; has one Texture response, but has two M– (Human Movement Minus) responses; seems tenser in this protocol; has more monster responses (poorer interpersonal relationships).
5B. *Post-therapy protocol*: A bit more of a rigid and defensive approach, but has more positive interactions between people and between animals; has better form quality.
6A. *Pre-therapy protocol*: Several morbid responses; poorer form quality; greater difficulty with the task as a whole; amorphous human percepts (ghosts, skeletons)—difficulty with interpersonal relationships.
6B. *Post-therapy protocol*: Has more conventional responses; more rigid, but not as loose in thinking; no morbid or aggressive responses.
7A. *Pre-therapy protocol*: So morbid; responses are of poor form quality.

7B. *Post-therapy protocol*: A bit of a manic quality (so many responses); leads to perseveration? While this protocol shows some neediness and distress, it is less morbid and has better form quality than the other protocol; the subject really falls apart on the cards with color and affect.

8A. *Pre-therapy protocol*: More tension (Inanimate Movement, denoted as m).

8B. *Post-therapy protocol*: Emotional neediness; more able to see popular responses; overall form quality is better; greater complexity of responses (e.g., first two responses on the two protocols have the same content, but more complexity described in this protocol).

9A and 9B. 9B looks like and feels like the after-therapy protocol. The form quality is better; there is less reaction affect and color, but I am puzzled when I see that the D score is worse and Depression Index is higher than in the other protocol.

10A. *Pre-therapy protocol*: Very rigid and defensive protocol; lacks Human Movement and Texture responses; striking difficulty integrating to produce a Whole response.

10B. *Post-therapy protocol*: Less defended; no aggressive responses; two Texture responses and one Human Movement response; able to connect with another person; form quality improved; still striking difficulty integrating and giving a Whole response; ability to see pairs seems improved.

The results of the Rorschach blind interpretations were self-explanatory. Perhaps the most promising part of the interpretations was the fact that the interpreter was able to predict correctly in nine out of the ten sets of pre- and post-therapy test protocols which were given to her. This suggests that nine out of the ten subjects made enough improvements for Dr. Hutchinson to be able to discern the differences. Since Dr. Hutchinson was provided with the contents of all the protocols as well as with the Structural Summaries, the implication would be that the Rorschach contents helped depict the progress that the subjects made in therapy.

Teacher's Report Form

The TRF consisted of a teacher's ratings of the subject's academic performance and four adaptive characteristics (working hard, behaving appropriately, learning, happiness) in part one and of the same teacher's ratings of the subject on 118 specific problem items and two open-ended problem items in part two. The problem items were scored on a three-step response scale—zero, one, and two—similar to the one used in the Child Behavioral Checklist (Achenbach, 1991). The results of the TRF will be presented in two tables.

In Table 4.7, the summary of the problem scales in terms of *Number of*

Table 4.7 TRF: problem scales

Subjects	No. of items		Total score		Total T		Internalizing		INT T		Externalizing		EXT T	
	Pre	Post	Pre	Post	Pre	Post	Pre	Post	Pre	Post	Pre	Post	Pre	Post
1	4	19	4	20	46	51	1	11	49	60	1	3	52	54
2	12	18	12	18	51	55	2	7	46	57	4	3	55	54
3	9	9	9	11	49	52	4	7	52	57	0	0	42	42
4	36	36	59	53	63	62	9	2	59	46	42	42	76*	76*
5	3	19	3	21	43	57	1	5	43	53	1	5	49	56
6	37	23	51	27	66	57	13	9	63	59	24	15	70*	64
7	36	67	49	96	65	75*	3	12	51	62	18	38	67	78*
8	4	8	6	12	45	51	0	2	37	46	1	3	52	54
9	59	71	78	90	72*	75*	13	20	63	67	17	29	66	73*
10	3	9	3	9	43	49	1	9	43	50	1	7	52	58

* clinically significant

Items, Total Score, Total T, Internalizing, INT T, Externalizing, EXT T will be presented. The specific problems will not be presented due to the low number of subjects. The variables were defined as:

1 *Number of Items* represents all of the items that the teacher identified as problem items for a subject.
2 *The Total Score* represents the total of the score based on the three-step response scale—zero, one, and two, which the teacher had endorsed on the aforementioned problem items.
3 *Total T-Score* represents the T-score based on the total score. Achenbach suggested T-scores between sixty-seven and seventy as borderline and T-scores above seventy as clinically significant. He further divided the syndrome scales into two blot categories: *Internalizing* and *Externalizing*. The syndrome scales designated as Withdrawn, Somatic Complaints, and Anxious-Depressed are grouped under the heading of *Internalizing*, whereas the syndrome scales designated as Delinquent Behavior and Aggressive Behavior are grouped under the heading of *Externalizing*. He noted that these groups of problems have been called Personality Problems versus Conduct Problems, Internalizing versus Externalizing, Inhibition versus Aggression, and Overcontrolled versus Undercontrolled.
4 *INT T* and *EXT T* represent the T-scores for *Internalizing* and *Externalizing* respectively. The scores of specific syndromes will not be presented here due to the low number of subjects.

The results from this part of the study were the most ambiguous. Improvement was demonstrated in one subject's *EXT T*-score (Subject 6), whereas deterioration was shown in two of the subjects' *EXT T*-scores

(Subjects 7, 9). In addition, Subject 7's *Total T*-score exhibited significant deterioration.

In Table 4.8, all of the subjects' Academic and Adaptive Scores will be presented.

The results of the academic and adaptive scores were mixed. No significant gains were noted with the exception of Subject 6. In perusing the forms, I discovered that six out of the ten teachers had known the subject they were evaluating for one to two months during the pre-therapy testing. Theoretically, the teachers did not know the subjects well enough to rate them. Some of the teachers omitted numerous items at the pre-therapy level, which significantly decreased the number of subjects who could have their pre- and post-therapy scores compared. Moreover, the pre- and post-therapy ratings of one subject (Subject 10) were filled out by different teachers. All of these factors may have contributed to the complication of this test's outcome. Yet another factor which may have added to the decline in the teachers' ratings of the subjects was the closing of the school. The teachers and the students were troubled by the news, and there was much chaos caused by the news. The teachers could have been more distressed and not as effective in controlling the students' behavior, or the teachers could have been projecting their own feelings onto the students. The teachers may not have been as effective in their teaching performances, either. Thus, the students' problematic behaviors might have been likely to increase, whereas their academic performances might have been just as likely to decrease.

House-Tree-Person drawings

As previously indicated, the HTP drawings were blindly interpreted by Dr. Driscoll. She was asked to predict which set of drawing was pre-therapy

Table 4.8 Academic and adaptive scores

Subjects	Aca. perf.		Works hard		Beh. appr.		Learning		Happy		Sum	
	Pre	Post	Pre	Post	Pre	Post	Pre	Post	Pre	Post	Pre	Post
1	4.50	4.50	—	5	—	5	—	5	—	4	—	19
2	3.00	3.00	—	4	—	3	—	4	—	1*	—	12
3	3.00	2.67*	—	5	—	7	—	5	—	3*	—	20
4	3.67	4.00	4	2*	1*	1*	4	4	1*	3*	10*	10*
5	3.00	3.00	5	3*	4	3*	5	4	4	2*	18	12*
6	3.17	3.83	2*	5	4	4	4	4	3*	4	13*	17
7	2.83	2.67*	4	2*	2*	2*	4	3*	4	2*	14*	9*
8	2.67*	2.33*	—	5	—	3*	—	3*	—	5	—	16
9	1.50*	1.50*	1*	1*	2*	2*	1*	1*	4	3*	8*	7*
10	3.50	3.00	6	3*	6	3*	6	4	7	4	25	14*

* means clinically significant
— no rating was provided by the teacher

and which was post-therapy for each subject. The subjects will be identified as 1A (pre) and 1B (post), and so forth; her interpretations of their drawings are included as well. Dr. Driscoll correctly predicted nine out of the ten subjects' sets of drawings. Subject 10 was the only exception. The results of her interpretations were as follows:

1A. *Pre-therapy*: Considerable emotional energy invested; in a turmoil, turmoil is very tied into what's happening in the family; some wish fulfillment? Anxiety, feeling out of control, afraid, vulnerable, obviously preoccupied with father; impulsive, pressured; preoccupied with aggression.

1B. *Post-therapy*: Some insecurity, need for grounding; some barrenness, loss, untapped potential? Much calmer, more contained than in the other set; if this is post-therapy, loss may be related to father? Still deprived-looking, but better than the other set of drawings.

2A and 2B: A lot of similarity between the two sets; somewhat reserved, a little guarded; has internal strength, but lacking in direction.

2B. *Post-therapy*: Appears to be somewhat healthier; more willing to interact and connect with people; more willing to trust.

3A. *Pre-therapy*: Tentative, unsure of self, deprivation, loss in family? Confused feelings; need of nurturance, dependence, support; warmth within; threatened by outer world?

3B. *Post-therapy*: More confident, less anxious, but still has some sense of insecurity.

4A. *Pre-therapy*: More developmentally-immature than the other set; strong dependency needs; strong orientation toward the outer world, toward other people; high achievement needs; learning disabled? Some anxiety; positive affect covering underlying fears.

4B. *Post-therapy*: Dependency needs are strong; some anxiety, oversensitivity; more mature-looking than the other set; calmer, more control; "person"—more mature, more human; lots of emotional energy (trying too hard?); a hysteroid quality?

5A. *Pre-therapy*: The drawing in this set looks more aroused, engaged than in the other set; more effort; younger, more dependent, very preoccupied with details, almost compulsive; one can "feel" the child more than in the other set; very concerned with family issues; a secret of some kind; tentative about interpersonal relationships? Sexualized female drawing—is this an issue?

5B. *Post-therapy*: Much more contained and less revealing than the other set; more emotional control; still some sense of insecurity and insignificance; more reality-based.

6A. *Pre-therapy*: Anxious, vulnerable, guarded, not very open to interpersonal relationships; sad, dysphoric, insecure.

6B. *Post-therapy*: Also guarded regarding interpersonal relationships, but a more stable-looking set of pictures; not revealing as much; still signs of instability and problems.
7A. *Pre-therapy*: Much emotion focused on family; more anxiety than in the other set; striving; extroverted.
7B. *Post-therapy*: Some sadness (less anxiety); ambivalent feelings regarding family; concerned with security and dependency; trauma in life somewhere; more psychic energy; high need for achievement.
8A. *Pre-therapy*: Guarded, cautious about letting others in; inner self very vulnerable, susceptible to damage or wounds; need for warmth; need to protect him/herself.
8B. *Post-therapy*: Very ambivalent about letting others get close concerning social/interpersonal relationships; does family depend on him or her (parentified or overresponsible child?); dependency needs, but also aggressive impulses or orientation; inner self still confused, but much better-looking (less wounded) that in the other set of drawings.
9A. *Pre-therapy*: Peculiar quality to drawings; sadness; poor integration of feelings and cognition.
9B. *Post-therapy*: Looks like progress has been made, but still anxious, odd; more interaction with the world and people; less isolated-looking; more growth potential.
10A. *Post-therapy*: More ambitious drawings; taking on a challenge; cautious about openness with others; dependency needs important; complex feeling about family.
10B. *Pre-therapy*: Some confusion of feelings, direction; some anxiety.

Similar to the Rorschach's blind interpretations, the rater for the House-Tree-Person drawings correctly picked (blindly) nine out of ten sets of pre- and post-therapy drawings. These results excited me because, like the Rorschach results, the H-T-P drawings may have reflected true inner changes which occurred in the subjects. Even though the outer behavior may not have demonstrated much change, it is possible that the therapeutic change transpired at a deeper level. These inner changes will be more likely to stay with the subjects and have positive impact on their futures than if the changes were more behavioral in nature.

Therapists' reports

Each therapist was asked to note the important information and the changes which occurred with her subject throughout the process. They provided me with the following notes:

Subject 1

In the fall of 1992, when this subject began sandplay therapy, she seemed sad and withdrawn, exhibiting little affect and energy. As the therapy year progressed, the subject became more and more animated, outgoing, and energetic. Her self-confidence and self-esteem seemed to significantly increase. Towards the end of therapy and the school year, she regressed slightly due to the probability of having to testify for the second time in the murder trial of a close relative. Overall, this subject showed significant growth in her sense of well-being.

Subject 2

This subject is very quiet and reserved, cautious, and a good student. She has physical problems such as scoliosis, and she wears a brace. She has problems socially—not taking responsibility and having disagreements with others. The feedback from the school social worker is that this subject bloomed socially this year. This subject spent the year developing a trusting relationship with me. She never opened up much verbally, but she became more open in her play and less worried about failure. I think her major accomplishment was developing this trust as she is very scared of making herself vulnerable.

Subject 3

Her parents divorced, and her father has been in and out of the home. When he's there, he lives in a separate bedroom. He takes thirty-plus pills of medication every day (he had four heart attacks, and he has kidney trouble). Throughout the year, this subject became more assertive, more willing to express herself (she is basically a very shy person). At a group meeting, she bravely revealed her sexual victimization. At one point, she considered testifying against the perpetrator who brutally sexually assaulted her numerous times a few years back. Ultimately, she decided not to testify because she could not recall details of the assaults. This subject developed a very positive transference with the therapist. She was very interested in completing the sandplay process. The positive changes I see were her assertiveness, her ability to trust, and her willingness to confront the darkness.

Subject 4

This subject was taken out of his mother's home by the Child Protection Agency when he was two. I suspected that he was an early neglect and, possibly, abuse victim. He lives with his two sisters and their grandmother. His grandmother recently took in an infant foster child. The school social worker was concerned about the impact of this change on the subject. The subject's many sand pictures depicted primitive fighting scenes. Changes were seen in his ability to be more focused (he was all over the place when he first started, very restless), some resolution of his inner struggles concerning good and bad, and his ability to trust and connect. He was very connected to his therapist.

Subject 5

This subject's mother is actively chemically dependent. At one point, the school social worker was very concerned about the subject's welfare (she was late for school, often unkempt, and, at times, very sick or tired). This subject changed from more of a caretaker (to her mother) to more of a needy child. She was more willing to show her needs, more willing to relate, and to accept help. At the end of the therapy, her mother reportedly decided to enter a chemical dependency treatment program. This subject was very happy about her mother's decision; however, the subject was very sad because she did not know where she would be going to school (this school would be closed) the next year.

Subject 6

This subject was extremely needy (the best description would be to say that she was a bottomless pit), very stubborn, very demanding, almost in a compulsive manner. During the first few sessions, she would tend to use up all of the color glues, all of the stickers, etc., and she would still appear to feel empty. After working through a negative transference that occurred when her therapist set some limits, the subject settled down and was willing to work through her issues. Some improvement was shown in her willingness to share, to trust, and to connect. At the time of termination, she still seemed like she had a long way to go. However, she was less unhappy, more content, and friendlier.

Subject 7

Initially, she was very scattered in her thinking and in her play. Improvement was noted in her ability to focus longer on an activity. This subject was guarded about discussing family problems after she was returned to her mother and appeared to have increasing problems in the classroom at the same time. She stated pleasure at being involved in sandplay therapy. She was able to build a warm relationship with this therapist. The subject was very spiritual.

Subject 8

This is a very vivacious, lively child. She was referred due to violence in her home. She has trouble with reading. Her mother is reportedly supportive and quite competent. The changes in the subject over the year were as follows: more able to stay on task; not as easily overwhelmed; more able to concentrate; less overwhelmed with thoughts and fantasies of threat and violence; more able to play openly; more creative in her artwork. In addition, her self-confidence increased.

Subject 9

This subject has difficulty in expressing her thoughts. She needs help processing information. She appeared to be more grounded at the end of therapy. She was extremely upset about the closing of the school when she first learned of it, but she appeared to have worked through some of the grief and loss. She was guarded about family issues.

Subject 10

This subject began sandplay enthusiastically, eager to participate. She made good progress in her therapy, being able to express the conflicts in her life in the sand tray. As boundaries were set, however, she became less enthusiastic and slightly sullen. In January, the subject's mother raised the issue of trust and a misunderstanding concerning the taking of pictures, along with the possibility of the school's file reflecting her being involved in therapy. A conference was held with the mother, and the issues were resolved with her. However, the subject became protective and defensive in the remaining sessions. I believe she finished the work that she needed to do and was ready to leave therapy as early as February. The closing of the school was difficult for her, and she said she wanted to spend her time in the classroom. She did not want to miss out on classroom activities while attending sandplay sessions. Her feelings were further heightened by the terminal illness of her teacher with whom she was very close. The subject did not complete all twenty sessions; she terminated after the eighteenth session.

The therapists' reports are basically subjective and not represented in any objective rating form. However, the author feels that since each therapist knew her subjects most intimately, she was in the best position to evaluate what had transpired in each therapeutic process. The reports were based on twenty successive sessions that the therapists had with all of the children (except for Subject 10, as noted above). Therefore, the therapists were able to observe the qualitative changes that occurred in addition to the pre- and post-therapy quantitative scores. Each therapist's description of each subject's progress was self-explanatory. Essentially, the therapists observed positive changes in each child, although the changes occurred in different ways. The author could see unique changes in each of her own four subjects, but felt that there were general positive changes that could apply equally to all of them. For example, they became more assertive and less aggressive, more flexible and less rigid, more trusting, open, and integrated.

Limitations of the study

As Strupp (1973) pointed out in his psychotherapy outcome studies, increasing attention is being paid to the variables in the client's life situation and environmental factors. One important factor which was totally unexpected and which appeared to greatly impact this study was the announcement of the closing of the school, which occurred in the middle of the study, and the eventual closing of the school. This school was the center of the children's lives, especially the children in this study. It is possible, given some of the children's significant difficulties, that if it were not for this school, some of the children in this study might have needed to have been placed in a residential setting.

When the announcement of the closing of the school occurred, one of the subjects told me that her classmates and her teacher cried for an hour. While the same subject was progressing beautifully on her sandplay work during that session, she made a tray which had a "big hand which ate people, and other hands which scared people." This subject began by making a large hole in the middle of the sand. Then she firmly placed a large green hand in the hole and added sand around the hand. Then she stated, "I want more hands." She used the fingers of the hands to scratch in the sand tray, indicating, "There are all kinds of dead people with hands left." She noted that the big hand liked to eat people and, "Who's next?" She found a man with a gun and buried him in the ground with only his head showing. She said, "There," meaning that she was done and that the man was killed.

The same subject made another picture which she labeled "A town of houses" towards the end of the study. Among the "houses" she chose was a school. She announced that the school was buried because a hurricane came. She also stated that there was a big volcano that grew angry because it was snowing really hard. The volcano exploded. As a result, all houses, including the school, were buried way down. She said, "You may not be able to find all of the houses because they are buried." In this tray, there was not much to see because the houses were under the sand. One of the houses she buried was a red house with a white roof that she identified as the school. The rest of the houses she chose were "a teepee, a Chinese house, and a space needle."

On the same day that the news of the school's closing was announced, another subject made a sand picture which I labeled "Save the school." She poured a lot of water in the middle of the tray and made a big mound. Then she embedded a large cross in the front of the mound. She added a preacher on top of the mound with a cat and a dog sitting by him. Then she smoothed out the area in front of the mound and wrote, "Save _____ [the school's name]." Around the mound gathered many people, mostly children.

The closing of the school had a great impact on the teachers as well as on the children. I had contact with some of these teachers and knew that they strongly believed in providing a special educational environment for minority children. When their beliefs were shattered and their careers placed on hold, they also suffered a great deal along with the children. The teachers' suffering was likely to impact their interactions with the children in the classrooms. Consequently, the teachers' ratings of the children were likely to have been influenced as well.

The closing of the school also affected the therapists. While all of the therapists were devastated by the news, the impact was twofold for the author. Initially, the author felt distressed for the children and for the school staff. She also was discouraged since the news might have erased the therapeutic progress which had been made up until that point. While these children might have been used to having doors shut on them, this news came quite unexpectedly. All the therapists could do was to hold the children's hands and help them deal with the grief. It was not an easy task to pick up the pieces when the damage was done somewhat deliberately and by a human organization.

Another unexpected event occurred in the middle of this study. The therapists' supervisor encountered illness, which resulted in an operation. As a result, regular supervision did not happen as smoothly as planned. This interruption in the supervision may have had some mild adverse effects on the effectiveness of the therapists. However, Ms. Weller resumed supervision immediately after her discharge from the hospital, therefore minimizing the possible harmful consequences.

All of the therapists were beginning sandplay therapists, which may have been another important variable. Even though they were under the supervision of a qualified therapist, they might have made more avoidable mistakes. The author admits to making mistakes which probably would not have been made in the hands of an experienced therapist. Consequently, if the therapists in this study had been more experienced, the outcome might have been different, and most likely better.

As indicated in the Psychotherapy Outcome Research section, Strupp (1973) pointed out the importance of the therapist variable. His studies showed that the personality attributes and attitude of the therapist played an important role in the therapeutic outcome. In this study, this factor was not explored. Perhaps in the future, this research could be expanded to include the analysis of data in this area.

Similarly, this study did not analyze the individual differences among the subjects. Some of the subjects chose not to use sandplay much at all, and a few of the subjects appeared to be too emotionally immature to participate meaningfully in the sandplay process. For the latter cases, floor games were introduced. Floor games, invented by Nessie Bayley, were games which the therapist would play with the child on the floor, making use of miniatures and storytelling.

Subject 10 did not complete twenty sessions of sandplay; she stopped after the eighteenth session. An expansion of this study might involve excluding some of the subjects, e. g., Subject 10. Due to the relatively small number of subjects in this study, this idea was not feasible. Another minor criticism of this study had to do with the assignment of three subjects from the same classroom to two of the therapists. The two subjects who were treated by the same therapist appeared to be, at times, competing for attention from the therapist. The third subject, who was assigned to another therapist, appeared to feel left out and demanded attention from the aforementioned therapist. While this might seem like a minor problem, it would be advisable to avoid a similar situation in future research designs.

Another concern with this study was the use of one rater for the blind interpretations of all the Rorschach inkblots and one rater for the blind interpretations of all the House-Tree-Person drawings. If it is at all possible, using more than one rater for each test and averaging their findings would provide better and more objective data. Should this be done in the future, inter-rater reliability is a factor which needs to be considered.

Another important limitation of this study was its lack of generalizability. The subjects were mostly minority children who were high risk and from a small, parochial school. It is likely that the relatively successful outcome may not be applicable to children from a different setting such as a white, middle-class, public school. On the other hand, it may also be possible that the outcome would be even more successful with the latter population.

Another factor that should not be discounted was the maturation of the children that would naturally occur over six months, which was the length of the sandplay process. However, in light of the fact that these children came from extremely deprived backgrounds and that they continued to live in very adverse environments, their mental well-being would have likely deteriorated without any therapeutic intervention. Therefore, any gain they accrued over the six months has to be at least partially attributed to the therapy in which they participated.

Recommendations for future research

Here are some recommendations for conducting similar research in the future:

1 *The use of a control group:* By using a control group, the therapist can ascertain with more confidence that the favorable outcome can be attributed to the therapeutic variable, provided that significant difference is discovered between the two groups.
2 *The use of more homogeneous therapists:* This would help to reduce the possible uneven outcomes attributed to the therapist variable.
3 *Better selection of subjects:* Subjects who may not be appropriate for out-patient therapy, such as the psychotic children, should be excluded

from the study. Another selection criterion concerns the subjects' age. I think that, in this population, children 9 years old and older are better subjects because they are more likely to engage in the sandplay process.

4   *Better assignment of the subjects to a therapist.* If at all possible, it is preferable not to assign two children from the same class to the same therapist.

5   *Better use of the Teacher's Report Form:* For pre-therapy measures, it is important to find a teacher who has known the subject for at least six to nine months prior to the therapy. Another alternative is to employ the Parent's Checklist. However, with the population in this study, it was difficult to accomplish this feat.

6   *The separation of the roles of therapist and evaluator:* It is preferable that the pre- and post-therapy measures are conducted by a single independent evaluator. This would help to provide more objective data.

7   *A larger sample:* A larger sample would provide a broader database for objective analysis.

8   *A longer duration of therapy and/or some follow-up:* Subjects with the amount of damage that these children were exhibiting at the pre-therapy level would normally require a longer duration of therapy to reconstruct their personalities. Therefore, if a researcher with a similar study would extend the number of sessions or the length of therapy to at least twice the time, s/he would most likely obtain better results. Moreover, a follow-up of the subjects in this study may provide interesting results. I hypothesize that their adaptive behavioral changes may manifest in the future.

Chapter 5

Conclusion

The processes and outcomes of twenty sessions of sandplay therapy for each of ten elementary-school children were studied. The subjects were identified by the school social worker as the children who most needed mental health services. Pre- and post-therapy assessments included the Children Depression Inventory, Rorschach (Exner Method), Teacher's Report Form, and House-Tree-Person drawings. In addition, all of the therapists were asked to report on the changes they saw in their subjects.

On the Children Depression Inventory, marked gain was demonstrated for two out of the three subjects who showed clinically significant depression during pre-therapy. Six out of the seven subjects who endorsed the suicidal item at a pre-therapy level improved in their responses as well. On the Rorschach, improvement was seen in the cognition category of the structural summaries for at least eight of the ten subjects; in the categories of affect, self-perception, interpersonal perception and relations, and capacity for control and tolerance for stress, results were somewhat mixed. Improvement was noted in nine out of the ten Rorschach protocols as depicted by the blind interpretations.

The results of the Teacher's Report Form were ambiguous and showed no significant gains. Possible explanations for this phenomenon were offered. Nine out of the ten sets of the House-Tree-Person drawings revealed improvement as predicted by blind interpretations. Unique changes and progress were noted by the therapists in the therapists' reports for all of the subjects. Limiting factors which may have interfered with this study were discussed. Recommendations for future research were made.

As I approach the end of this study, I experience many mixed feelings. For one thing, I am deeply saddened that the twenty sessions of therapy with these children has come to an end. I feel strongly that further therapy is needed for all of the subjects in this study. At this point, since that is not an option, I only hope that the positive effects of the therapy will remain with each of them and help them cope with their futures of incredibly taxing difficulties.

As I was executing this project, especially during the time when I had to integrate all of the material, it struck me as a sandplay process in and of itself. The project was puzzling and mystical, as well as challenging and rewarding. The most satisfying moments occurred when Dr. Driscoll was able to correctly pick nine out of ten House-Tree-Person drawings and when Dr. Hutchinson was also able to pick nine out of ten sets of Rorschach protocols as post-therapy measures. While the more objective types of material produced mixed findings, the nonlinear, more qualitative forms of information provided decided results.

As I near the end of this part of my journey, I can confidently conclude that the integration of the art and the science of psychology can be accomplished. At the same time, I also realize that I must continue this journey; there is a need for similar research in the future, particularly to show that therapeutic changes can be reflected in the adaptive behavior of the subjects.

Part II

The author's sandplay case done in the United States

Chapter 6

Introduction of the case

Zana, an 11½-year-old Caucasian female, was one of the ten research subjects chosen for a sandplay therapy outcome study that was sponsored by the Minnesota Sandplay Therapy Group. The selected site of this study was a small, parochial school located in the inner-city of the Twin Cities. This school had about one hundred children with 90 percent of them being students of color. The subjects were chosen by the school social worker, who had close contact with every student in the school and knew which children needed mental health services the most. In the referral form, this school's social worker noted the following about Zana:

> This is an 11-year-old Caucasian female. She lives with both parents (they are, however, divorced and previously separated) and her older brother, age 13. She was the victim of repeated sexual abuse by a neighbor during the summer when she was 8 years old. The abuse involved intercourse and penetration with many objects; it was an awful account. The perpetrator was never prosecuted; he still lives next door, and she sees him outside all the time. Her father is chronically ill with a multitude of problems and is not expected to live much longer.

On one of the Teacher's Rating Forms, Zana was noted to be "nonassertive, not showing emotions, sad, friendly, honest, and kind."

As part of the research design, Zana was seen for an intake interview, a pre-therapy psychological assessment which included the administration of projective drawings, the Rorschach (Exner Method), and the Children's Depression Inventory. After the completion of twenty therapy sessions, the same battery of psychological tests was re-administered to her. The initial testing was administered by the author, whereas the post-therapy assessment was conducted by another child psychologist.

During the initial interview, Zana presented herself as an intensely shy and nervous girl who hid her hands mostly in her sleeves. Physically, she was slightly chubby, prepubescent, and had freckles on her face. She told me she did not like her freckles because her brother would tease her about them. In regards to her family history, she told me that after her parents were married for thirteen years, they had divorced the previous summer. She indicated that her father had just had his fourth heart attack and also had kidney stones which were about the size of ping-pong balls. She seemed anxious about her father's health. In addition to her parents and her 13-year-old brother, her uncle (her father's brother) also lived in the home. She noted that her mother worked with computers for a major firm in the Twin Cities.

When asked to draw a house, Zana drew a three-story "abandoned house" which was undergoing reconstruction because it had been set on fire by an arsonist in the past. Her projective drawings as blindly interpreted by a psychologist suggested, "Tentative and unsure feelings, emotional deprivation, confused feelings, threatened by external world, need for nurturance, dependence and support." Her Rorschach protocol indicated the presence of a great deal of tension and turmoil. The CDI score of twenty-four was extremely high. Children who obtain such a high score are known to be severely depressed and need immediate and intensive mental health assistance.

During the initial assessment, Zana was also asked to do a Kinetic Family Drawing. Upon being instructed to draw every family member including herself involved in some kind of action, she drew a big television with antennas in the middle of the paper, and the small heads of her aunt, uncle, mom, dad, her brother, and herself at the bottom of the paper. She drew her face at the lower left corner, farthest away from everything. Then she wrote, "We are watching TV" in very large print, occupying the upper half of the paper. Such drawings suggested very little movement and interaction in the family and that she was rather alienated from others and perhaps had a very low self-image.

During this assessment, Zana was clearly informed about the conditions of participating in the study, which included the completion of twenty therapy sessions of forty minutes each. She was told that she might choose to participate in any activity that she preferred. The activities included talking, playing a game, playing with toys, painting, drawing, sculpting, and sandplay. Zana was very eager in every session, participated fully, and made the most of her time. Frequently, she made one or two trays, did some painting, and did clay work or art design (using stickers). With the exception of one session that fell on her birthday, which we celebrated by having a party, and one other session in which she talked a lot and diligently did her first painting, she made one or two sand trays every session. For a total of twenty sessions, she made twenty-four trays; eight paint, crayon, and chalk pictures; four sticker art designs; and four clay sculptures.

Exposing confidential information is a very courageous and risky act. At this moment, I ask you, the reader, to hold Zana in your heart to keep her safe, and to give her your thanks as well as blessings.

Chapter 7

Zana's sandplay process
Recovery from sexual trauma

Sand picture 1

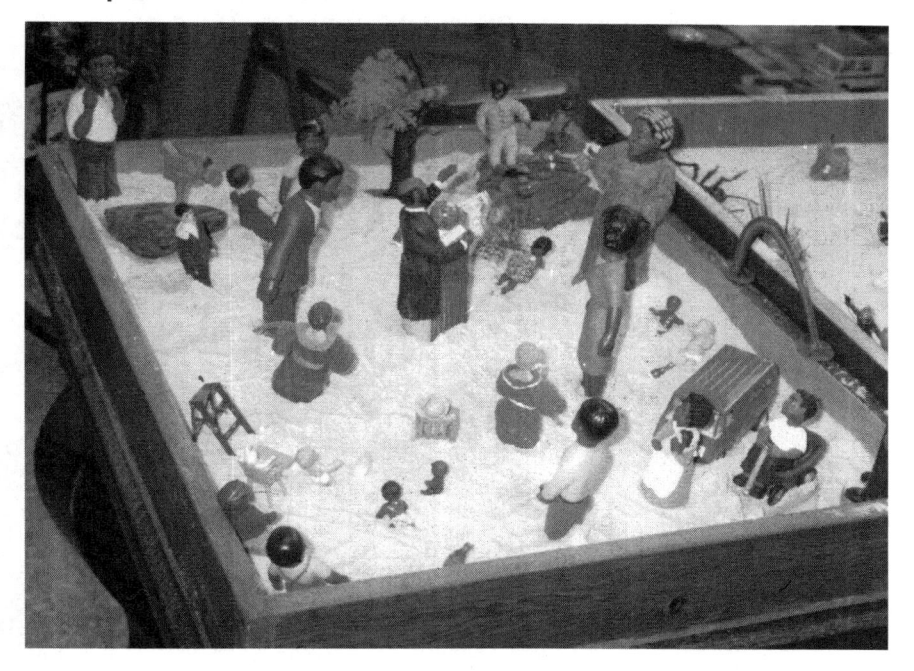

Figure 7.1 The initial searching.

Sand tray making process

After slowly smoothing the sand in the wet tray with both hands, Zana carefully picked out items for this tray (Figure 7.1). She diligently worked from all directions with intensity, seeming to have a center in mind.

The items she placed in the tray were in the following order: a black teenage boy in the upper right corner; a black couple (a male in a brown suit and a female in a purple dress) facing each other; an older lady with curls on her head; a little boy and dog in a wagon (lower right corner); a black policeman who ended up in the lower right corner (not seen in this picture, originally placed in the upper left corner); a pair of black children (a male in a yellow shirt and a female in a yellow dress) facing each other; a white girl in a blue dress near the black girl in the yellow dress; a little black male in a yellow shirt and blue jumper and a little white female in a blue top (lower left corner); a white male in a light brown robe with a blue neckline and a blue belt near the black man in a brown suit; a white female in a red robe near the black female in the purple dress; a green van near the boy in the wagon; seven babies in total, including a baby with a bottle nearby, a baby in a potty chair, and a baby in a high chair; a white female toddler with long blond hair and a little black toddler in a red printed dress near the large woodpile; a white male adult who ended up behind the black male in the brown suit (originally placed between the black couple); two green bottles including a wine bottle by two of the babies; two young black teens sitting on top of a natural pile of wood and rocks; a young black female adult wearing an apron and carrying a baby in her arms, near the van; an oak tree with leaves on only one side of the tree, facing the middle; a pizza in a box (mostly buried in the sand) and two bottles near the woodpile; a camera placed upon another woodpile (upper left corner); an adult black male in a white shirt with a child on his back (upper left corner); a rainbow sitting on the ledge of the tray, positioned between the two trays; a broomstick (not seen in this picture) in the hand of the black boy in the yellow; a red stepladder near the baby in the high chair.

After placing all the above items in the tray, Zana moved and rearranged several of the figures near the center away from the center, then smoothed the sand in the middle, placed a minister with a podium with a Bible on top of it right in the center of the tray. Then, she placed a miniature blue globe on top of the Bible, completing the tray.

Zana's comments

After completing the tray, Zana said:

> All these people get together and the preacher is preaching, saying that we should all be getting along, there should be no prejudice. He is preaching how we shouldn't fight and should not be racist. He had this miniature globe here, preaching, saying how the world should all get along. That guy there [the adult black male in the white shirt with the child on his shoulders] videotaped everything.

Therapist's interpretations

After an initial brief chat, Zana immediately walked over to the sandplay area and started to work. She was completely absorbed in the work, almost as if she were in a trance. Items were placed in a spiral fashion from outside of the tray towards the center. This circular fashion, along with the last item she placed in the center (the globe) appeared to represent her search for the psyche center of herself. Both the circle and the globe may signify wholeness (Cooper, 1979, pp. 36 and 74). In her opening statement, Zana seemed to be saying: "I need to find the inner wholeness, the inner peace."

The first item Zana placed in the tray was a child. Moreover, she placed a large number of children and babies in this tray. Children are symbolic of a beginning and of abundant possibilities (Matthews, 1986, p. 37), or the embodiment of potentialities (Cooper, 1979, p. 35). Children also represent innocence and simplicity (Cooper, 1979, p. 35). Jung, in explaining the psychology of the child archetype, stated that the "child" is all that is abandoned and exposed and at the same time divinely powerful; the insignificant, dubious beginning, and the triumphal end (Jung, 1968, p. 179).

The fact that Zana devoted so much energy to placing many children into this tray suggests that she was searching for possible potential change and perhaps the triumphal end. In addition, it may also represent her mourning for her lost innocence due to the past sexual abuse. Her damaged self seemed to be vividly demonstrated in the barren oak tree which was the only tree she placed in this tray. Even though the oak tree is a symbol of strength, durability, and courage, this oak tree had very few leaves and many bare branches.

Nurturance appeared to be present in the form of food—the pizza in a box, the baby bottle as well as other bottles. Upon closer inspection, of the four bottles, two of them were wine bottles. Could there be alcohol abuse in the family? Who among the family members were abusing alcohol and might be presenting problems? A check with the social worker revealed that Zana's uncle, who lived in the house, was an alcoholic and unemployed. Moreover, Zana's father had a history of abusing alcohol and quit drinking when he became sick several years ago.

The need for protection and a sense of vigilance seem to be represented by the figure of the policeman in the corner of the tray and by Zana saying that "the man" was videotaping the event. However, is the protection strong enough or adequate? Zana and her family members had an unfortunate experience with the police. Apparently, after they reported the sexual abuse to the police, the police lost the file and the perpetrator did not get prosecuted. How would all this affect Zana's self-image and her emerging femininity?

Another issue Zana seemed to be struggling with concerned the union of the opposites. She meticulously placed a few pairs of couples with a male facing a female, black next to white, and this represented her striving to integrate the polarities. Moreover, the story that she gave regarding the preaching of no prejudice and no racism by the preacher reinforced this issue.

As a Caucasian girl who lived in a predominantly black and Native American environment, both in her school and in her neighborhood, Zana appeared more comfortable identifying with blacks, as shown in this first tray. While it is understandable that Zana felt more comfortable aligning herself with blacks as suggested by this picture and other pictures that followed, I wonder how alienated she felt as a white minority in this environment.

While the whole tray seems to represent Zana's desperate need for help and her desire to reach inner peace and wholeness, Zana's strength is suggested by these objects: a green van; a wagon; a broomstick; a rainbow; and a stepladder. Both the van and wagon are means of transportation and capable of moving if they are placed on the right track. They represent potential resourceful energy. A broomstick, which is placed in a little boy's hand, represents magical power (Biedermann, 1989, p. 50) and the strength that can repel evil influences (Walker, 1988, p. 123).

Both the ladder and the rainbow are bridges, symbols of connection and communication between heaven and earth, or going from "the unreal to the real, from darkness to light, from death to immortality" (Matthews, 1986, pp. 113 and 155; see also Cooper, 1979, pp. 94 and 136). In addition, the rainbow is known to be associated with God's forgiveness and His covenant with humanity (Fontana, 1994, p. 115). The fact that Zana placed the rainbow on the ledge of the tray and the ladder far away from people suggests that these bridges are not well contained and cannot be readily accessible at this point.

The last item that she placed in this tray was a preacher. This preacher could represent what Jung designated the archetype of the old wise man. Edinger indicated that this archetype is a spiritual guide, a bringer of wisdom and healing, and a personification of the ego–Self axis (Edinger, 1992, p. 118). Could this preacher, the old wise man, help Zana heal the wound and repair the damage, i.e., ego–Self alienation that was caused by the sexual abuse and confusing racial issues? Perhaps Zana viewed me—the therapist—as the preacher, the wise old man who was going to accompany her through the painful and challenging journey of finding her inner peace and wholeness.

Overall, throughout this first tray, Zana appeared to be conveying not only her problems and issues to me, but also her strengths, her vulnerabilities, and her willingness as well as her courage to face her challenges in this journey of her psyche.

Sand picture 2

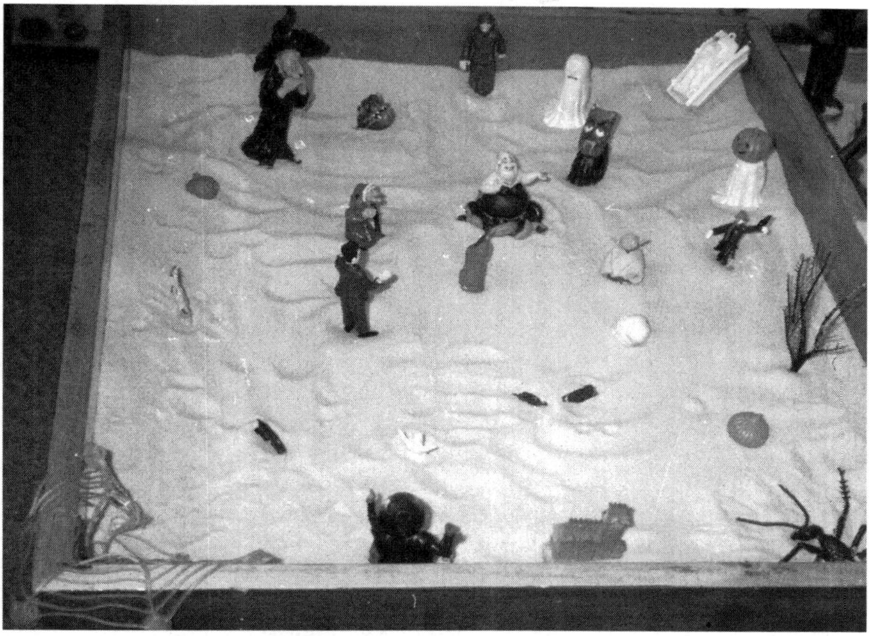

Figure 7.2 Down to the shadowy land.

Sand tray making process

After completing Sand Picture 1 and after being informed that there were five minutes left in the session, Zana immediately went to work in the dry tray. Similar to the way she placed the items in Figure 7.1, she worked in a circular fashion from the outside of the tray towards the center (Figure 7.2). The items she placed were in the following order: a spider web (lower left corner); a giant ant (lower right corner); a witch (upper left corner); a white coffin with a skeleton figure inside and with the lid open (upper right corner); two pumpkins and a pumpkin-head ghost; a black cat (the small black item nearest to the spider web); another witch near the spider web; a scarecrow ghost near the pumpkin-head ghost; a coral leaf; a hand (in the middle of the left side of the tray); a grim reaper (middle top); a white ghost near the white coffin; a blue haunted house (mid lower); a small white ghost; a colorful—red and blue—mask and a green-masked ghost; Yoda (to the left of the center) and a gnome with a red hat; a white skull near Yoda; two little black skeletons near the skull; the sea witch, Ursula; a Frankenstein figure across from Yoda; and a green finger with a red nail in the center of the tray.

Zana's comments

After finishing this tray, Zana said: "Giant witch is coming out of the finger." "Spider is growing bigger, making more webs." "Lady's hand is dead." "This guy is opening this guy's casket."

Therapist's interpretations

Zana apparently used up all the ghosts and witches that we had in the cabinet. Without a doubt, Zana immediately descended into the unconscious dark land. The similar circular or centering motion of making a tray starting from the outside and moving towards the inside suggests that she is reaching for the inner part of the psyche, perhaps again searching for that inner peace or wholeness.

The spider web, the first item that she placed in this tray, is a reminder that this is a dangerous journey of the soul (Cooper, 1979, p. 190). Although Zana appeared plagued by anxiety, she was willing to face the shadows—the skeletons and monsters of her life. Things seemed to be very gloomy; ghosts and deadly scenes were prevalent images. Her statements about the giant witch, the spider web, and the dead hand also mirrored the depressive atmosphere.

Significantly, her comment about the coffin ("This guy is opening this guy's casket") shed some positive light. The coffin, the mystic womb of the second birth, may represent redemption, resurrection, salvation (Cooper, 1979, p. 39), and the hope of rebirth (Walker, 1988, p. 129). Perhaps, Zana was making a statement about her willingness to work on her redemption and rebirth.

Moreover, positive forces are present and are represented by several figures in this tray. First of all, Yoda, the teacher or mentor of Luke Skywalker is placed near the center of the tray. Will this vulnerable, yet very wise figure be able to provide power and wisdom for Zana on her journey? Also, the coral (leaf)—the sea tree of the Mother Goddess; the moon, giver of life; the fertility of the waters (Cooper, 1979, p. 42) are present in this tray. A giant ant located at the lower right is another source of positive power. This diligent insect is known to be a helper of the divinity who created the world (Biedermann, 1989, p. 14). Zana, having similar characteristics of diligence and industriousness, appeared to be working hard towards self-transformation.

Sand picture 3

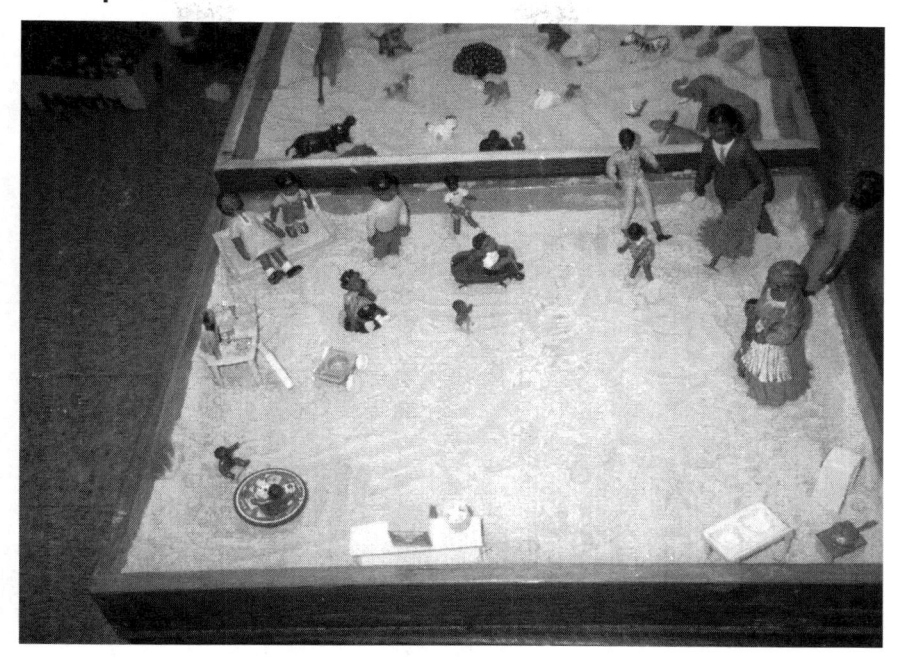

Figure 7.3 Grandmother is visiting!

Sand tray making process

A black couple (upper right corner), a grandmother with a child hanging on to her apron, a teenage boy (upper right corner), and ten additional children including three babies were present in this sand picture (Figure 7.3). One child was sitting on a wagon with a dog sitting behind him. Another child was talking on the phone. A baby was sitting on top of a picnic table (lower left corner). All of the people were African American. Furniture present in this scene was: a blue couch (upper left corner); a light blue dining table next to the couch; a blue potty chair in front of the dining table; a picnic table (lower left corner); an entertainment cabinet with a television and a lamp sitting on top (lower middle); a sink, a stove with a pot on it, and a refrigerator (lower right). On the top of the dining table, there were two bottles of wine, a can of beer, a pitcher and two cups, plates, knives, forks, and spoons. An unopened box of pizza was next to the dining table. There was a small pine tree standing in front of the adult black couple. Tracks were observed in the empty space (middle of the tray).

Zana's comments

After completing this scene, Zana gave the following story:

> It's Christmas time. Grandmother is visiting. There is a Christmas tree. The kids ordered a pizza and are watching TV. The little girl is talking on the phone and is saying, "Grandmother is visiting." The older kids are watching the younger kids. These two kids [babies] are drawing.

Therapist's interpretations

In the beginning of this session, Zana was told that her therapist would have to take a trip to Taiwan to attend her brother's funeral (his death was unexpected). Zana was shown the location on the globe where I was going. She was told that I would be gone for three weeks and that the next time we would see each other would be early December.

After this sharing, Zana was quiet; she showed no emotions. Then, she said, "I would like to do the sand." Similar to her approach in working on Figures 7.1 and 7.2, she worked from all directions and was completely immersed in this task. After placing the first item—a blue couch—in the sand, she placed the girl in the yellow dress on the couch in a lying down position.

In the subsequent review, Zana identified this girl as herself. The position that this girl is in indicates her passivity and alienation from other people, including family members. The other children are active, whereas she is the only one lying down. It is possible that the sexual abuse that occurred in the past has made her sad, mad, and/or angry. She is likely to feel unworthy, guilty, and unjustified. Perhaps she felt betrayed because her parents did not protect her. It may even be that she was angry at me for taking a trip and being gone for three weeks. While the scene she portrayed in this tray is a happy Christmas scene, she seemed alienated and did not actively participate in her environment.

Zana's current psychological state appears to reflect what Edinger calls the alienated ego (Edinger, 1992, pp. 37–61). In his attempt to explain alienation neurosis, Edinger states that an individual with such a neurosis is very dubious about his right to exist, has a profound sense of unworthiness, is scarcely able to act according to his best interests, and is cut off from a sense of meaning (Edinger, 1992, pp. 56–57). Zana's identification with the girl who is lying down resonates with the alienated ego description provided by Edinger.

Zana spent a vast amount of time in setting up the dining-room table. Such a meticulous act appears to be somewhat ritualistic, but could also signify her careful preparation for the upcoming soul journey. The pizza box remained unopened, but available for use. In addition, other kitchen items such as the sink, the stove, and the refrigerator were also available. While there seems to be a huge emptiness in the middle of her psyche as represented by the open space in the middle of the tray, her hesitant readiness to undertake the journey is reflected by the tracks that were crafted all over the empty space.

Similar to Figure 7.1, the children in this tray represent the beginning, abundant possibilities, and the potential for a bright future. Unlike the oak tree which was barren in Figure 7.1, the pine tree in this picture is very green and lush. This evergreen tree, though small, signifies uprightness, vitality, fertility, and immortality (Cooper, 1979, p. 131). Moreover, the presence of the pot which represents nourishment and the lamp which is a universal symbol of enlightenment (Walker, 1988, p. 143) suggests some optimism in her pursuit of this journey.

Sand picture 4

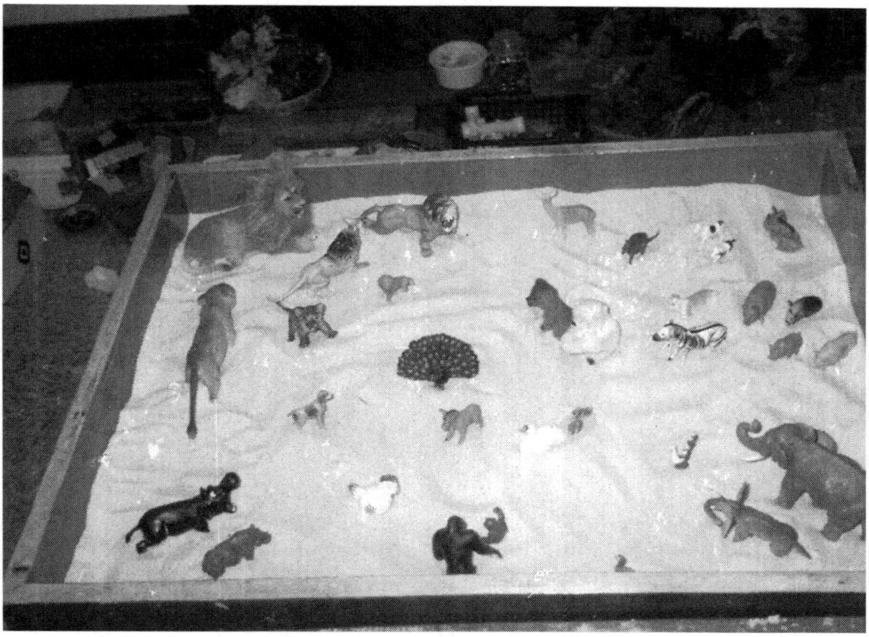

Figure 7.4 Animals are out.

Sand tray making process

After completing Figure 7.3, Zana was informed that there were fifteen minutes left in the session. She immediately walked to the dry tray and started to work (Figure 7.4). Again, she worked from the outside while moving towards the inside. In the upper left quadrant, she placed a lion family—four adult male lions including the large one with a mane, an adult female lion, and a lion cub. In the lower right quadrant, she put an elephant family (three elephants), a mother duck with ducklings, and a chicken. In the upper right quadrant, there were a rabbit family (three rabbits), two cows, a wild boar and three pigs, a dog, a zebra, a kangaroo (next to the cows), a deer and two bear cubs (one brown and one white). In the lower left quadrant, there were two hippos (one black and one brown), a chicken, a black adult gorilla and a brown baby gorilla, and a dog. In the middle of the tray stood a peacock, a donkey, and a mother swan with her babies.

Zana's comments

Zana, upon completing this tray, stated: "The zookeeper's car was getting towed. He told this guy to let out the animals. The zookeeper did not realize what he had done; now he has to collect all the animals."

Therapist's interpretations

On the way back to her class after finishing this sand picture, Zana told me that the previous night her dog, Mandy, was burned very badly. Apparently while cooking, her uncle accidentally dropped hot soup on the dog's back. Zana said that the dog cried badly last night and that the vet was going to check on the dog today. She was wondering whether the dog would live. This was the first time Zana had spontaneously shared emotional information about herself with me and marked the beginning of a positive transference.

For this tray, Zana placed the large lion in the upper left corner first. The lion, the king of the jungle, represents strength, power, courage, and fortitude (Cooper, 1979, p. 98). Most noteworthy is the number of lions she placed in the tray—a total of four male lions, a lioness, and a cub. Cooper noted that the lioness is an attribute of Tara—an earth and maternal symbol—whereas the lion cub represents a newly initiated Bodhisattva (Cooper, 1979, p. 98). While lions are generally known to be ferocious and possibly cruel, they seem to be rather peaceful and nonviolent in this scene. Perhaps Zana was trying to draw out her instinctual energy, the one which is strong and powerful, and yet nonviolent and compassionate.

Coming out of her depression, Zana seems to draw instinctual energy not only from the earth (lions, elephants, pigs, dogs, etc.), but also from the water (swans, hippos, ducks) and from the sky (the birds). Moreover, the transforming power, represented by the peacock, is located right in the middle of this tray. The peacock, known to eat most food on the ground, including possibly poisonous materials, can easily digest everything and make them beneficial for the body. The peacock is also a symbol of immortality (Fontana, 1994, p. 87). Additionally, its tail or "wheel" which contains many colors represents totality or wholeness (Matthews, 1986, p. 146). It seems evident that Zana was working towards transforming herself and achieving inner wholeness.

The last item that Zana placed in this tray was the donkey. The donkey is traditionally known to be associated with stupidity, patience, and obstinacy. It might be that this animal will guide Zana patiently through some of the mistakes that she may have foolishly made in the past. Might the donkey, the animal ridden by Jesus Christ when he entered Jerusalem, assist Zana in her spiritual journey?

Paint picture I

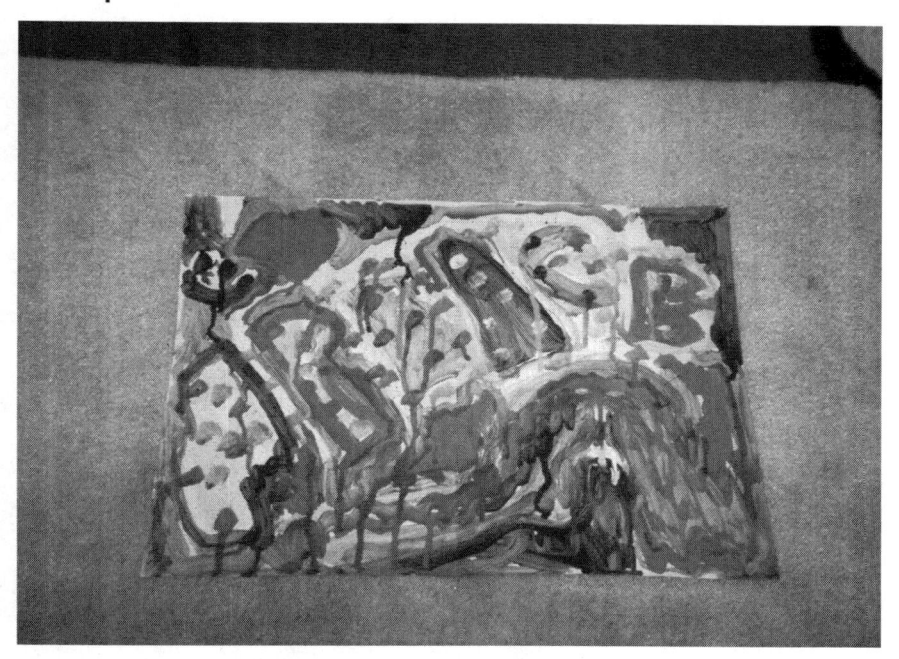

Figure 7.5 Peace?

Paint making process

Four weeks passed before I saw Zana on this date. She told me that her dog was okay and that the Thanksgiving holiday had gone well. Then she chose to paint.

In the middle of this picture which consisted of red, black, and green colors on a white and black background, Zana painted the word PEACE in the same colors (Figure 7.5). These letters were surrounded and covered with the same-colored dots which appear to be streaming down the surface of the painting.

Upon completing this paint picture, Zana was told there were ten minutes left in the session. She asked if there was anything else she hadn't done. I mentioned stickers. She went to work with the stickers and did a very colorful design of the stickers on both sides of a piece of paper which she then took home with her. She did not do a tray.

Zana's comments

While she was painting, Zana related in an agitated manner what appeared to be a very upsetting experience with the school basketball team. Zana stated that her mother had paid fifteen dollars for her to participate with the team. However, at her first practice, she got taken out for twelve minutes and thirty-six seconds, and during her second practice, she didn't get to play at all. When she complained to her mother about the basketball coach, her mother said there wasn't anything she could do. We discussed ways that Zana could handle the situation, and she seemed to calm down after the discussion.

Therapist's interpretations

This paint picture reflects Zana's emotional agitation, her anger, sadness, and her longing for inner peace. The anger is represented by the red color (de Vries, 1984, p. 383), whereas sadness and depression are reflected in the tear-like drops and the black background (Cooper, 1979, p. 39). Nevertheless, she displays positivity in her statement of "peace," painting boldly across the center of the paper and using green, which is known to be associated with the awakening of springtime and growth (de Vries, 1984, p. 226; Matthews, 1986, p. 91).

Sand picture 5

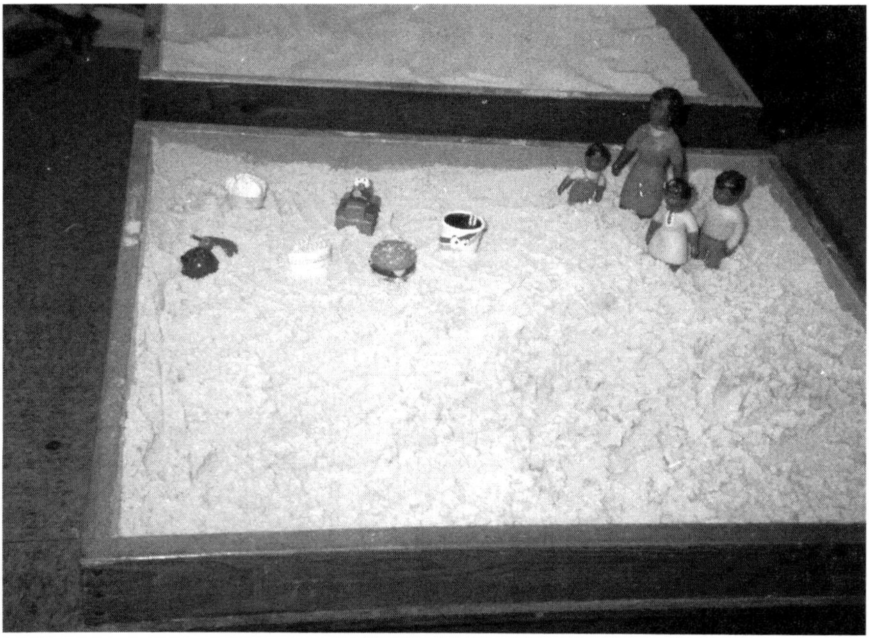

Figure 7.6 A family event.

Sand tray making process

In the upper left quadrant (Figure 7.6), there were a number of food products—including several McDonald's food items—a drink, a hamburger, French fries—an ice cream sandwich, an ice cream cone, an apple, and a pear. In the upper right quadrant, there was a black adult female and three black children. In the lower right quadrant, water was poured into the sand.

Zana's comments

Zana stated: "This is my mom, my brother, this is me, and this is my cousin. On Sunday, she always takes us out for breakfast, and on Saturday, for lunch."

Therapist's interpretations

At the beginning, I told Zana that I had brought new items (food items from McDonald's). She immediately used those items for this tray. This suggests her continuing positive transference with me.

The tray, however, seemed to remain at a conscious level as it depicted a regular ongoing family activity. Following her comments about the tray, Zana went on to share more of her family history—in particular, about her great-grandmother whom she called grandmother and who seemed to be a positive person for her, and about her father. She said her father had been very sick and had been in and out of the home. When he was at home, he would sleep in a separate bedroom from her mother (they are divorced).

Then, she talked about the situation with the basketball team. Apparently she decided to write a note to her coach to complain about her lack of playing time. Interestingly enough, she had more playing time after that and was happy about it. However, she was still a bit mad at her coach because her coach did not personally apologize to her. It was evident from this example that Zana was becoming more assertive and happier.

On this particular day, Zana took the water bucket and poured some water into the sand in the lower right quadrant. As she was pouring the water, she commented, "What happens when it gets wetter?" She used her hands to touch both the dry and wet sand, then examined the difference. An attempt on her part to compare, contrast, and unite the opposites (wet and dry) was taking place. Additionally, according to Edinger (1985, p. 47), water is thought of as the womb and *solutio* (the softening of the male ego in the feminine water) as a return to the womb for rebirth. Zana's watering sand act may signify a desire to return to the womb for rebirth.

Later in the session, Zana made a sticker design with two faces and stated that the two faces represent her brother and her cousin. She added, "It's boring to be the only girl (in the family)." An increasing awareness and concern about the masculine–feminine division as well as a need to have a balanced relationship between the masculinity and femininity in herself begins to emerge.

Sand picture 6

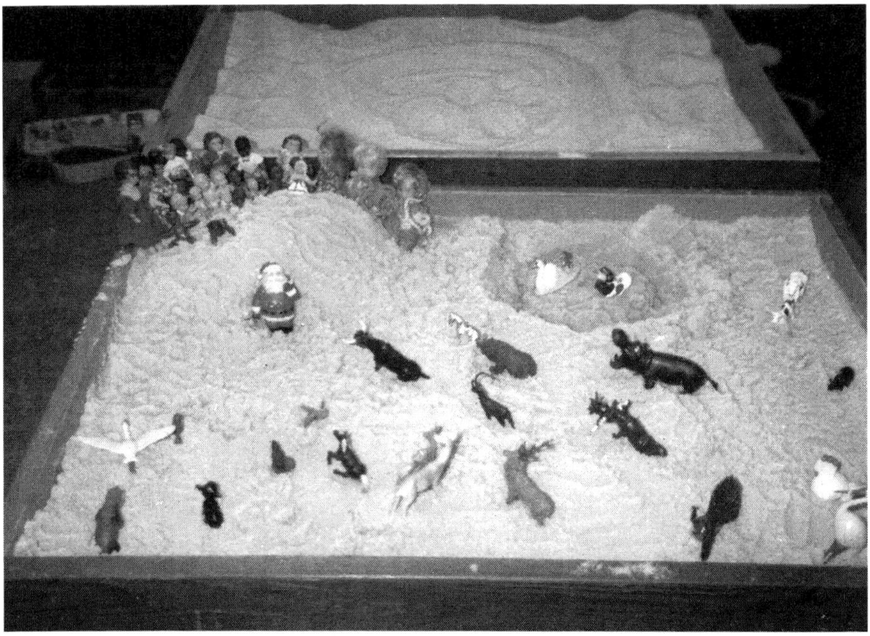

Figure 7.7 Children, Santa Claus, and animals.

Sand tray making process

On the mound, which is located in the upper left corner, there were twenty-three children including eleven babies (Figure 7.7). There were both white and black children. At the bottom of the mound, Santa Claus stood in between the children and the animals, which occupied the rest of the sand tray. In the upper mid section, Zana dug a little pond (sand circle) and a moat between the pond and the rest of the tray. In the pond, she placed a swan, her babies, and a duck. In the upper right, she put a couple of cows. In the lower right quadrant, there was a black cow (near the mid right edge of the tray), a black hippo, a black and white goat (near the black bull, only partly shown), a black bull, a peacock, a chicken, and a stork. In the lower left quadrant, Zana placed a seagull, a brown dog, a black lamb, two bluebirds, one blackbird, and a black horse. In the middle of the tray stood a black bull, a gold horse, a brown bear, a black goat, a mother and baby deer, and a stag (Zana called it an elk).

Zana's comments

Upon completion, Zana told this story:

This was the night before Christmas. All of the kids have gone to bed, dreaming about Santa Claus bringing presents in the morning. In the middle of the night when mom and dad had gone to bed, Santa woke the kids up and told them that children should share things with the animals. Then, all of the kids were getting ready to go. Santa told the big kids to help the little kids to get dressed. He took them to the forest; they went to the forest with him [Santa] on his sled. They got there, and the kids were afraid, so they stayed on top of the hill because of their fear. Santa Claus told them that if they weren't afraid of the animals, then the animals would not be afraid of them and would love them. All of the animals came running and flying in. They stopped; the kids were still afraid. Santa Claus told them that if they each chose one animal to love, the animal would return the love. This baby [the black baby in front] wanted to go and meet the elk, so the baby went up there and gave the elk the present—love. The rest of the kids did the same. Santa told them not to kill, shoot, or eat animals or kill creatures, but to preserve the animals. He added, "Therefore, when your kids grow up, they can enjoy and love animals, too."

Therapist's interpretations

Zana was immersed in making this tray. For the first time, she poured a lot of water into the tray to mold the mound and to wet the pond. When she completed this tray and told her story, both of us stood there in awe, not saying a word. It was an extremely moving moment, and I felt very numinous. We shared this wonderful moment together. Interestingly, at the end of this session, Zana was able to hug me comfortably in saying good-bye for Christmas vacation.

This is the first time that Zana made a mound in a tray. The mound is known to be a healing image and is associated with transformation (Reece, 1995). In addition, a circle was made next to the mound, again reflecting centering and transformation. As soon as Zana placed the Santa Claus figure in the center of the tray, seemingly as a bridge between the children and the animals, she made the circle. This phenomenon is consistent with one of the themes of a speech that Kay Bradway made at the 1995 National Sandplay Therapy Conference. Bradway pointed out that a tray evidencing the development of the transcendental function often followed a tray in which a bridge uniting opposites appeared. In this case, a circle which represents transcendental function occurred in the same tray after Zana placed a bridge symbol—the Santa Claus figure.

Significantly, the first thing that Zana did in the next tray that she made on the same day was to draw a circle. In an attempt on her part to integrate opposites, love versus fear, consciousness represented by the humans versus unconsciousness represented by the animals, a genuine transformation at her ego–Self axis seems to have taken place.

In this session, both Zana and I were transformed, and we knew it. Moreover, according to de Vries, Santa Claus (St. Nicholas) is known to be the patron saint of children, virgins, and the poor (de Vries, 1984, p. 340). It is likely that Zana was asking me as a Santa figure to help her heal from the trauma she received from the sexual abuse in her past. With the presence of what appears to a strong co-transference (Kay Bradway's term), healing and transformation begin.

Sand picture 7

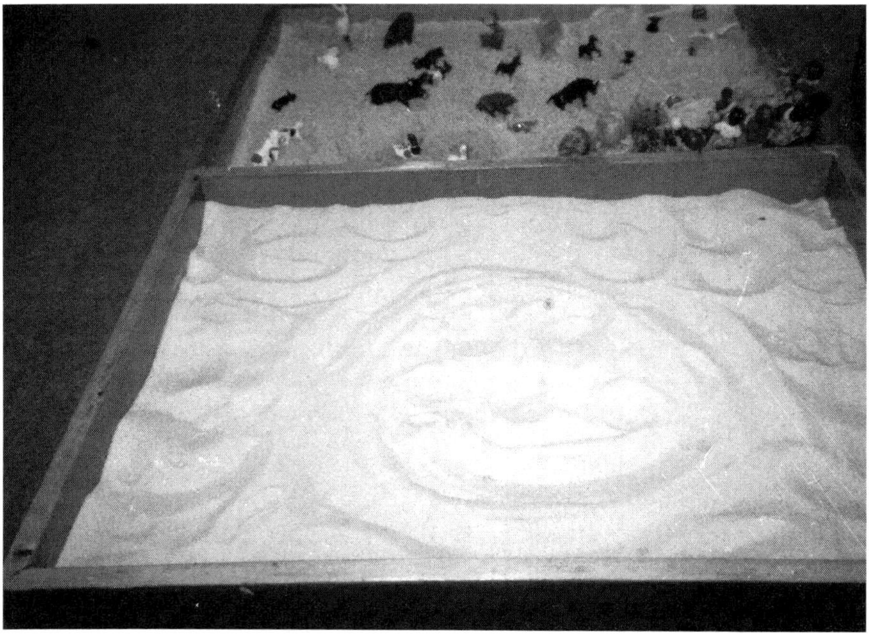

Figure 7.8 Black as a president?

Sand tray making process

When Zana found out that she had five minutes left, she walked to the dry sand tray and proceeded to draw a big circle with her finger (Figure 7.8). Then she added facial features and hair. Afterwards, she drew two little faces in each upper corner.

Zana's comments

This is Zana's story:

This is a man and these are two women over here [two upper corners]. This guy [the center figure] wants to be the president. He is black so he can't run. But the two women told him that he should become the president because that's what God wants him to be. Then Pope John Paul III came and said God told him no black should be the president. And the ladies got together, they were mad because he also said that no women should be priests. Pope John Paul III went home and thought about it, came back the next day and said, "God came and told me that there should be black people running for the president." These women settled down, happy that they got their way, but then they were wondering if a woman could be the pope.

Therapist's interpretations

As indicated in Figure 7.7, a centering occurred after the appearance of a "bridge"—which unites opposites. This picture seems to be reflecting Zana's first step toward the manifestation of the Self, as termed by Kalff (Kalff, 1980, p. 29). In addition, on another level, Zana appears to be making a transition from Kalff's animal-vegetative stage to the fighting stage (Kalff, 1980, pp. 32–33). Increasingly, Zana shows more self-confidence and assertiveness.

Sand picture 8

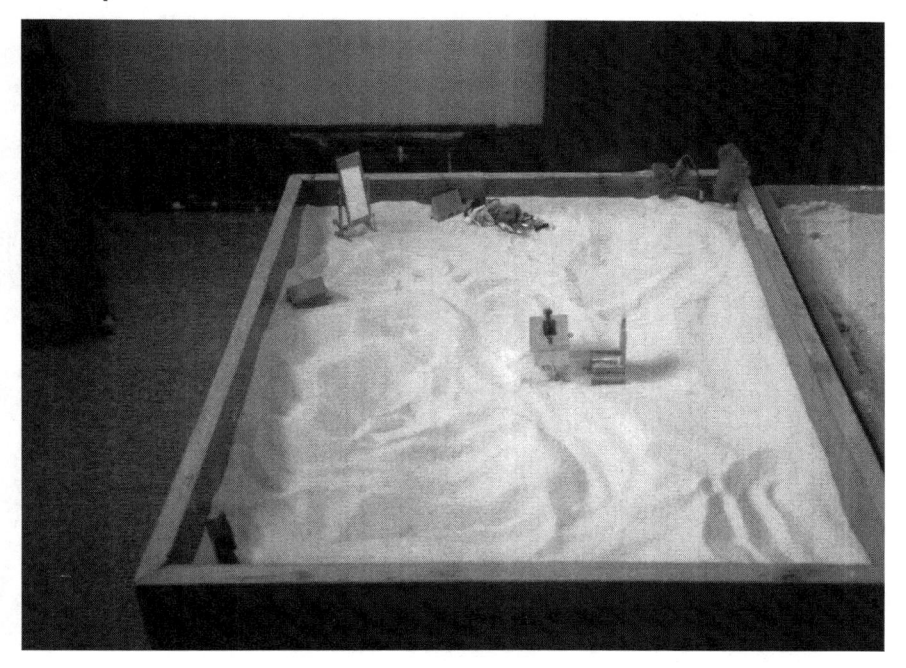

Figure 7.9 My room.

Sand tray making process

After finishing a hospital scene (picture omitted) in the wet tray, Zana made Figure 7.9 in the dry tray; she placed the items into the sand tray in the following order: a sewing machine and a golden throne (center); a standing mirror (upper left); a grandfather clock (lower left); a large red flower with a stem and a bud (upper right); a small dog in a red-colored doghouse (left middle); and a small blue dollhouse, an open treasure chest with three baby dolls in or near it, a red bicycle and a globe (upper middle). Then, Zana placed a picnic table in the tray before removing it.

Zana's comments

Upon finishing this tray, Zana stated, "This is what my room is like." Then she explained that her mom and dad were going to buy a sewing machine for her. She commented that the flower was the flower her father brought home from his work for her. She noted that she had a mirror, a globe, babies (dolls), and a tall clock in her room. Then she pointed out that the dog is her dog who liked to ruffle things up and crawl under things.

Therapist's interpretations

At first glance, this is a very bare picture. The golden throne that is placed in the middle of the tray has no one sitting on it. The sewing machine, located also in the middle, is standing alone. The mirror, a symbol of reflection and the examination of self, wisdom (de Vries, 1984, p. 323), and a soul-catcher (Walker, 1988, p. 145), placed in the upper left, reflects nothing.

Things appear somewhat gloomy. However, the fact that Zana was sharing the contents of her room with me seemed significant. She has invited me into her sacred place and perhaps is letting me know how empty she has felt inside. Towards the end of this session, Zana asked what miniatures she could bring to donate to the Minnesota Sandplay Therapy Group, the professional group that is providing the pro bono service to her and the school. In spite of the bareness that she seems to feel inside as suggested by this tray, she displays an eagerness to share. This reminds me of the poor widow who was praised by Jesus in the Gospel of Luke for her very small amount of offering (Chapter 21:1–4).

Sand picture 9

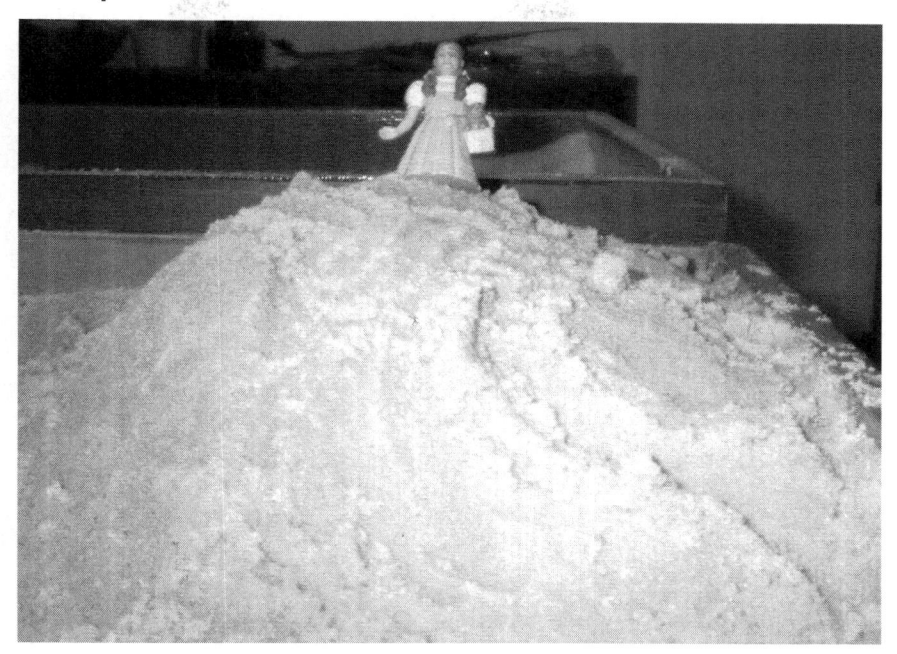

Figure 7.10 On top of the world.

Sand tray making process

After crafting a large mound in the upper right corner of the tray with trails going down the sides, Zana placed the Dorothy figure, the heroine of *The Wizard of Oz*, at the top of the mound (Figure 7.10). Dorothy carried a basket that contained her pet dog, Toto, in her hand.

Zana's comments

Zana said about this tray: "This is the world, and this is an ordinary girl. My grandmother often said that no matter what decision you make, if you think before you do it, you will be always on top. This girl is on top of the world."

Therapist's interpretations

This is the second mound that Zana has made during this sandplay journey. In creating the mound, she added more water to the wet tray in order to make the mound higher and more solid. When she was shaping the mound, she patted it very firmly and commented, "It is real solid." After smoothing out the mound, she carefully carved out the pathways down to the ground,

76 Author's sandplay case in the United States

Dorothy, a shy, introverted, and yet courageous girl, went through a horrendous journey and eventually found her way home. Zana, resembling Dorothy, appear to be standing at the beginning of a dangerous journey, ready to descend into the world. Is she truly ready to face the challenges? I should point out that this is the first time that Zana has identified herself as a white person in the sand trays.

Sand picture 10

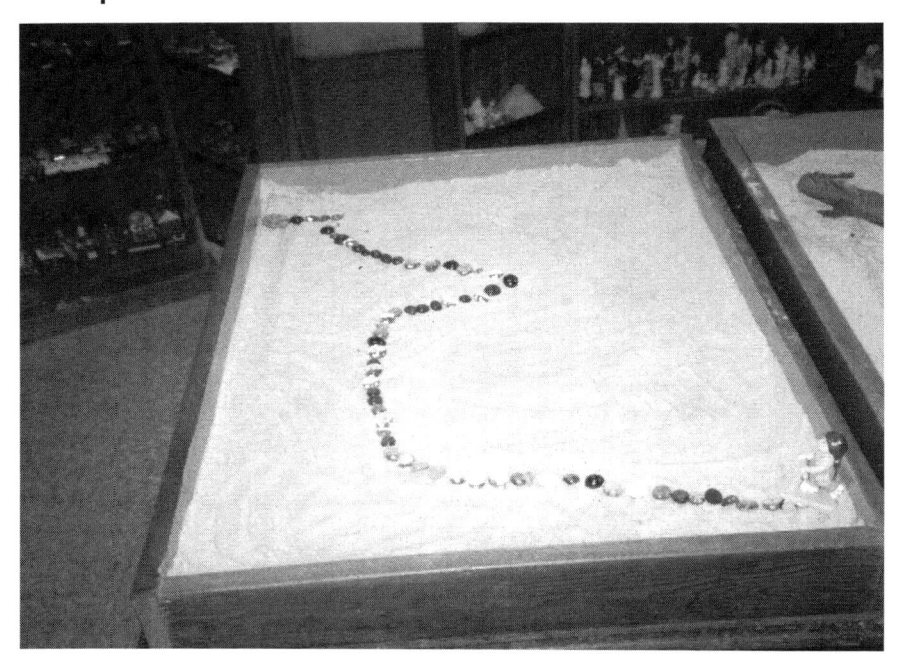

Figure 7.11 My journey.

Zana made two clay works, one prior to the making of this tray (Figure 7.11) and another one after the previous sand tray. These clay works were done on two different dates. They were of breakfast and dinner foods, including bacon, sausages, eggs, pancakes, pizza, drinks, and fruits.

Sand tray making process

Zana used different-colored flat glass marbles to build a path from the lower right corner to the upper left corner. A girl with ponytails in a jumpsuit and a pair of tennis shoes on a non-motorized four-wheeler was placed at the beginning of the path (lower right corner). She had one foot up in the air.

Zana's comments

Zana identified herself as the girl on the four-wheeler. She related the following story: "I go out to the world and this is my path [pointing to the glass-marbled path]. At this last place [pointing to the large glass marble at the end of the path], I stopped. If I like and want to live there, I'll live there."

Therapist's interpretations

Prior to this tray making, Zana did two clay works, both consisting of many food items. She carefully made them and seemed to be preparing to go on the upcoming soul journey. In building the path in this tray, Zana carefully chose different colored marbles and deliberately arranged them from the beginning to the end. The fact that she meticulously chose every marble reflects a certain amount of self-determination and self-assertion. She seemed rather confident that she could make choices concerning her life.

The girl that she chose for this journey looks about 5 or 6 years old, very confident, unafraid, and energetic. That is the age that Zana was before she was sexually molested by her neighbor. With the making of this tray, perhaps Zana is reclaiming the self-confidence that she had at her earlier age. When she was done, both Zana and I stood there looking at this tray in awe. It is a beautiful scene, and the light of her life appears to be shining.

Sand picture 11

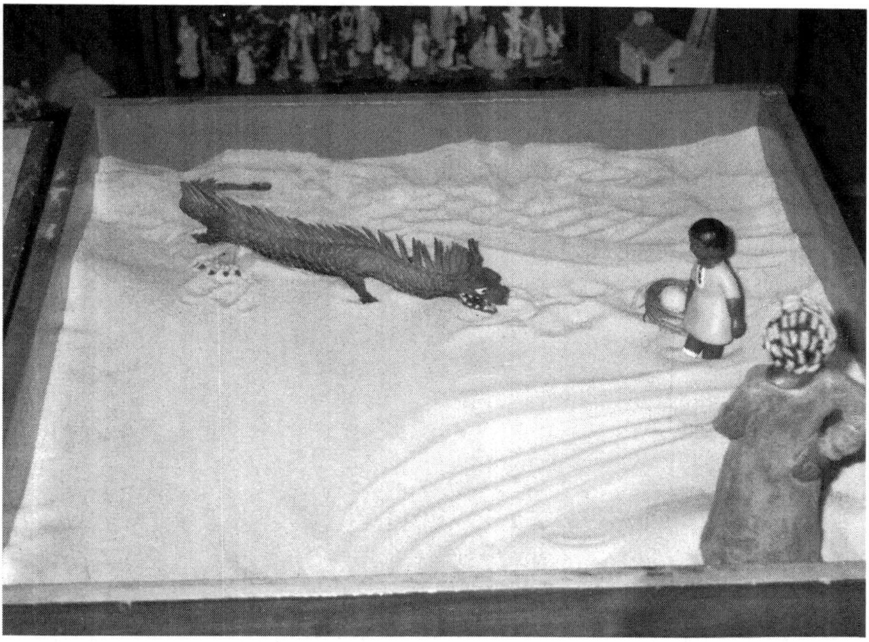

Figure 7.12 The demon.

Sand tray making process

A girl in a yellow dress was placed next to a basket with two eggs (one is blocked from view) and facing a dragon which resembled an Eastern dragon (Figure 7.12). A hand with red nails was placed near the lower right leg of the dragon. An older lady with her hair in rollers stood in the lower right corner of the tray on a small mound. Tracks were visible between the older lady and the little girl and next to the dragon in the upper right quadrant of the tray.

Zana's comments

This is Zana's story:

> This girl was having a bad dream. A demon was coming behind her, and its nest of eggs was by her. She was looking at the eggs and saw the demon. Her hand got caught in the nest. Then there was a voice. This lady was telling the little girl that she could control her own dream, that her arm could be freed, and that she could go to the demon, the demon will help her find her way home.

When Zana was asked about the hand, she replied, "[It belongs to the] people who didn't control the dream. They're afraid of the demon. He killed them and ate them."

Therapist's interpretations

After making the clay work (the dinner one) and Figure 7.11, Zana was told that there were five minutes left. She immediately went to work and made Figure 7.12. Her selection of the dragon was very shocking to me because I, after a long period of debate, had just chosen the dragon as the subject of my symbol study. This felt like what Jung would call synchronicity, a meaningful coincidence.

Moreover, I was amazed by the fact that Zana succinctly described the contradictory characteristics of the dragon: benevolence versus destruction. In Eastern Asia when one mentions the dragon, the following images would most likely emerge: benevolent, beautiful, friendly, wisdom, genius of strength and goodness, luck, fortune, fortitude, spirit of change, powerful and transforming, angels, loving, and anything associated with the emperor. In the Western world, the images and words associated with the dragon are quite the opposite. They might include: evil, terror, destructive, ugly, nasty, mean, gruesome, terrible, terrifying, monstrous, dangerous and disgusting. Western dragons are also known to spread diseases and plagues, to have poisoned fangs, and to be murderers (Hong, 1994).

Zana called this dragon a "demon" and stated that the girl was having a bad dream. It is possible that the dragon symbolizes the monstrous sexual abuse that she had encountered in the past. Zana clearly stated that her hand was caught in the nest which contained the dragon eggs. She seemed to indicate that she had inadvertently gotten into this ordeal and was afraid to face this shadow side of herself. Perhaps with my help, represented by the lady in the rollers and by the voice, Zana could face the demon, could confront the sexual abuse, and could be free from its bondage. At the end of this session, I shared with Zana the contrast between the Eastern and Western dragons and a story of a benevolent Eastern dragon.

Sand picture 12

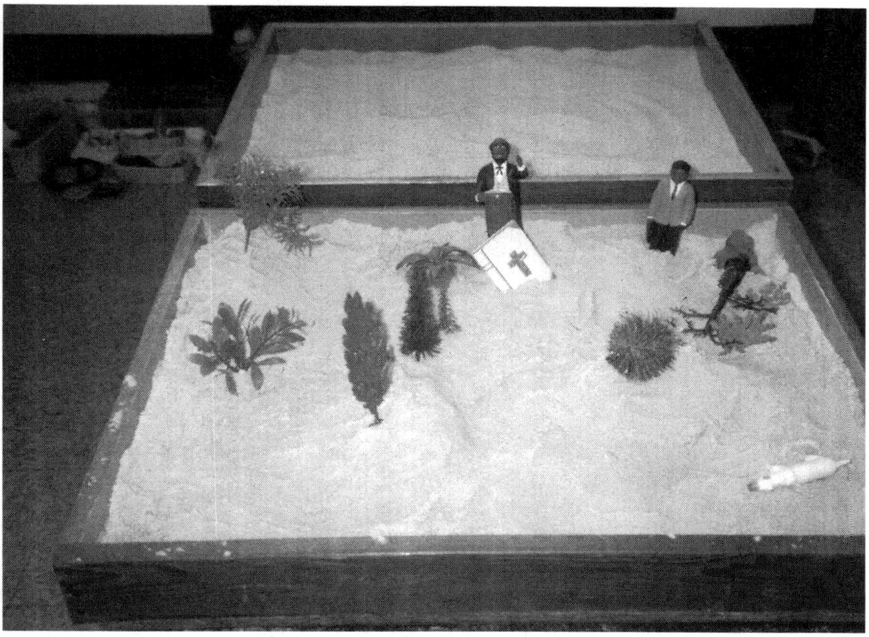

Figure 7.13 The destruction.

Prior to this tray (Figure 7.13) and in a previous session, Zana made a beautiful and serene Maya village, right after I shared with her about my trip to Mexico where I visited a Mayan village.

Sand tray making process

During the brief chat Zana and I had at the beginning of this session, Zana related her troubled feelings about school. In particular, she was angry at her teacher, who Zana felt had wrongfully accused her of inviting a friend to school who threatened other students. In addition, Zana was deeply troubled by the news that her mother's job was in danger. Zana stated that the machine might take over her mother's job.

In contrast to the last serene scene that she had made, this time Zana created a rather devastating scene. Two trees were placed on the right side of the tray, lying down on the ground. One of the trees downed was the barren oak tree seen in Figure 7.1. A dead bluebird was next to the oak tree, and a dead polar bear was on the ground as well. A black man in a business suit holding a briefcase was standing near the downed trees. The preacher with a podium in front of him, also appearing in Figure 7.1, was placed in the upper middle of the tray. A huge Bible was placed in front of the podium.

Zana's comments

Upon completing this tray (Figure 7.13), Zana said, "This man [the businessman] here wants to construct a building. He is cutting down the forest. The preacher is telling God to forgive him." She emphasized, "This man [the businessman] wants a building, so he is cutting down the forest and killing the animals."

Therapist's interpretations

Both the trees that perhaps represent the life force (de Vries, 1984, p. 473) and the mother polar bear that usually symbolizes the fearless and courageous mother who is ready to defend her cubs (Walker, 1988, p. 363) on the right side of the tray are down and dead, whereas the trees on the left side are alive and well. The contrast between them suggests a polarity in the psyche. The very noticeable difference between the two men, a peaceful preacher and a troublemaking businessman, further reinforces the notion of this personality split.

Significantly, the preacher and the Bible, which has an inscription of a cross on its cover, stand right in the middle (top) of the tray, suggesting that the possibility of reconciliation and integration in regard to the psyche polarity is likely to take place, especially in view of the fact that the cross is known to have a capacity to connect the horizontal and the vertical planes (Cooper, 1979, p. 45).

Sand picture 13

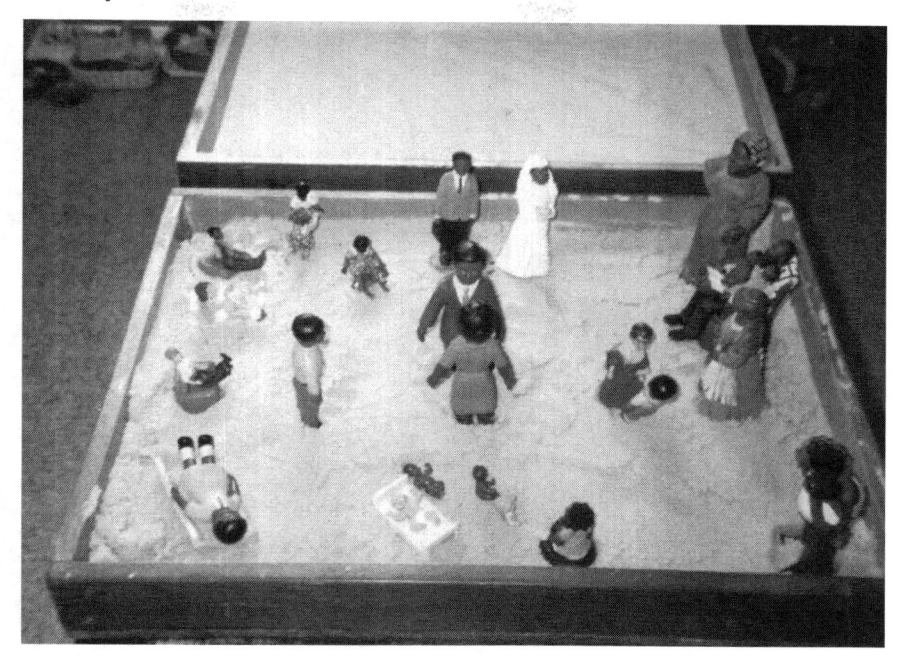

Figure 7.14 The wedding.

Sand tray making process

Zana produced the following scene (Figure 7.14). The black man in the business suit holding the suitcase was standing next to the bride, who was facing away slightly. The adult black parents were placed in the middle of the tray facing each other. The woman in rollers was put in the upper right corner. Next to this woman was a grandfather figure with two children on his lap, reading a book. Next to the grandfather was the grandmother figure with a child hanging on to her apron. In the lower right corner was a black father with a child on his back.

Many children were scattered around the tray, including two pairs consisting of a white female child and a black male child facing each other. Three children were sitting on chairs, whereas a girl in a yellow dress was lying down on a flat couch. Four babies were present (two black and two white), with one lying in a baby's crib. Next to the four babies was a black girl sitting on a chair, talking on a telephone. A girl in a red-printed dress sitting on a rocking horse was placed to the left of the bride and groom. A black boy in a yellow shirt was standing, facing the direction of the parental couple.

Zana's comments

This is Zana's description of the scene: "These two [the bride and the groom] are getting married. All these people are coming to the wedding. Most people are standing. This lady [the one in rollers] is watching, and this one [the grandfather figure] is reading stories."

Therapist's interpretations

In this wedding, the bride seems to be facing away from the groom, and most of the people do not seem to be actively participating in this event. Many pairs are present and facing each other in this tray. The combination of a seemingly inactive wedding and many interacting couples suggests a great divorce between the psyche's parts—one part that desires to join in, and another part that is ambivalent.

Even more significantly, the girl in the yellow dress who subsequently was identified by Zana as herself is lying down on a couch. This lack of interest in participation seems to indicate that even though the theme of the union of opposites or what the alchemists called *coniunctio* is taking place, Zana has very ambivalent feelings about the process.

Sand picture 14

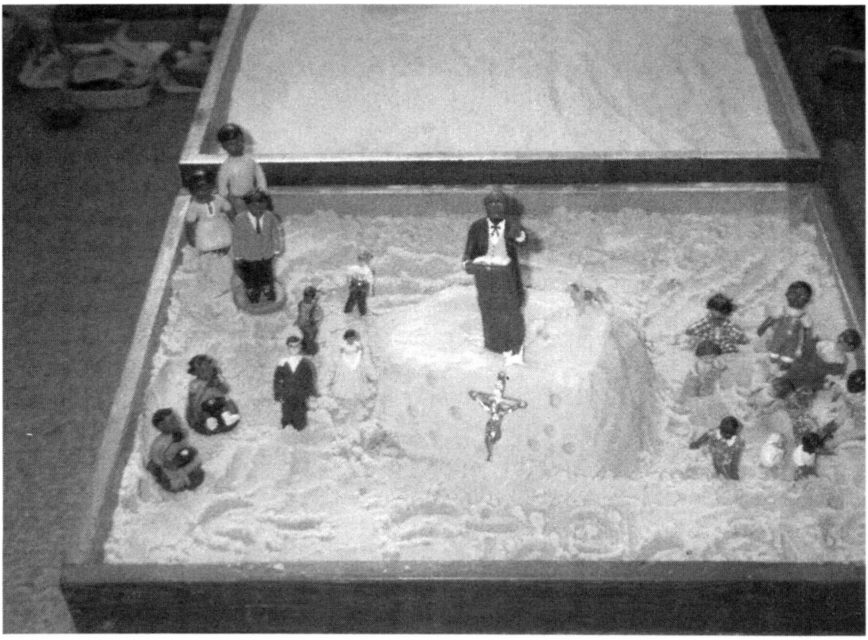

Figure 7.15 Save the school.

Sand tray making process

On this date, the decision by the Catholic authority to close down this school was announced. In the past, efforts have been made by numerous people, including all the therapists involved in the therapy project, to try to save the school. However, the efforts were to no avail, and the bad news arrived on this date. Zana heard the news for the first time. She, along with all the other children in this research group, was extremely upset about the news. After a short discussion about the school closing, she made this tray (Figure 7.15).

On top of a solid, square mound molded in the center, a preacher, standing behind a podium (also present in Figure 7.1 and 7.12), was placed. A small white cat and a dog were beside him. On the front side of the mound, Zana dug out eight small holes and placed a cross with a Jesus Christ figure in the center. To the right side of the mound, she placed nine children and a collie dog. To the left side of the mound, she put two children in yellow outfits; the black man in the business suit; a white child and a black child standing beside a white adult male and a black adult female; a female black child talking on a phone, and a male black child also talking on a phone. In front of the mound (lower center of the tray), these words were engraved, "Save _____ [the school's name]."

Zana's comments

She said: "This is a priest. He wanted Archbishop _____ [the archbishop's name] to reopen the school. All these people are saying that he should keep the school open."

Therapist's interpretations

This school that was very firmly crafted in the center of a square mound has been a solid ground for Zana for about five years. The ground or the earth symbolizes static perfection, immutability, integration, as well as permanence and stability (Cooper, 1979, pp. 157–158). The preacher, an old wise figure, adds a measure of stability because of his firm standing and wise preaching. Psychologically speaking, this centering theme may symbolize the inner searching for stability and strength in Zana's psyche.

Windows are known to symbolize gateways to air, light, knowledge, and vision (de Vries, 1984, p. 502). In this tray, eight windows of the school are present. Eight is a perfect number and an expression of wholeness (Edinger, 1985, p. 71). Thus, a tendency on Zana's part to seek further understanding and enlightenment of self and to reach for inner wholeness is evident.

The cross with the Jesus figure in front of the school building is also very centered and prominent. In a Christian sense, symbolically, the cross signifies transcendence of grave difficulties (death) and a chance for rebirth (resurrection). As a therapist, I wonder if this cross represents Zana's urge for redemption from the tribulation of sexual assaults.

Interestingly, while this sand picture displays Zana's superficial despair and agitation toward the closing of the school, it also reflects, in a deeper sense, the continuation of her attempts to transcend herself and to arrive at an inner wholeness.

Sand picture 15

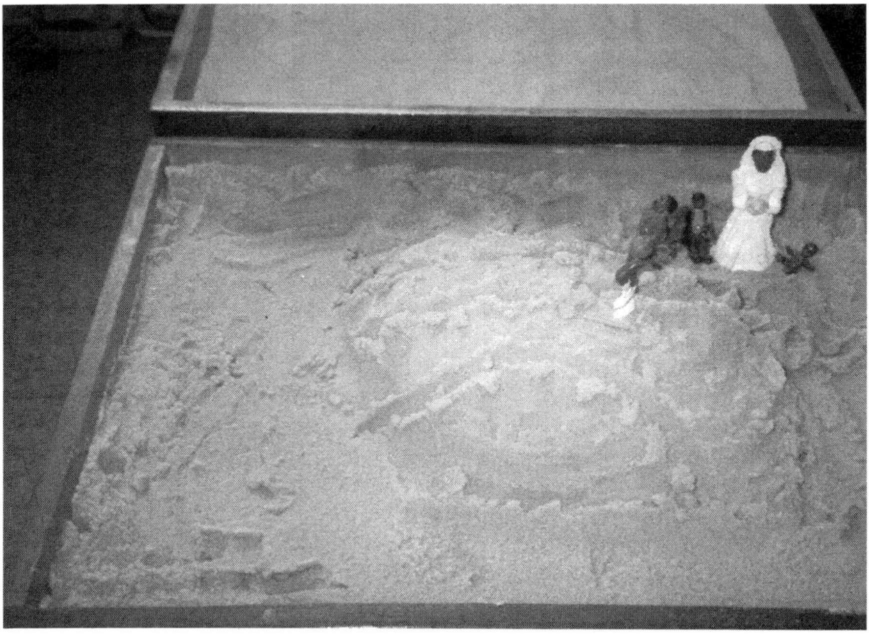

Figure 7.16 They are marrying.

Sand tray making process

This tray was made a week after Zana received the news about the school closing; she was still very unhappy about the news. She stated that she was very upset because, "It's discriminating against poor people." It is well known that this school was set up to help educate inner-city, underprivileged children. The closing of it seems to reverse the good will that was demonstrated initially by the Catholic authority.

After the initial brief chat, Zana immediately went to work in the sand (Figure 7.16). After pouring a lot of water in the tray and molding a large mound, she patted all around the top surface to make it smooth before carving the tracks. Next, she surveyed all the cabinets, picked out the girl with the yellow dress, and placed her on top of the mound. Shortly afterwards, she replaced the girl with a very muscular basketball player who had one foot up in the air and one hand holding a basketball. To the side of the mound in the upper right corner, there was a bride, a child, and a baby. All the people in this tray were black.

Zana's comments

As she completed the tray, Zana said: "This is a big basketball [the mound], and he is going to marry her [the bride]. She and the two kids are watching him. They are going to get married."

Therapist's interpretations

In contrast to the previous marriage scene (Figure 7.14), where the bride was facing away from the groom, here the bride is watching the groom intensely, and they are going to be married (Zana said). This active marrying scene appears to be truly a union of opposites or *coniunctio* as coined by Jung. It is essential and a fundamental step toward individuation.

Zana solidified this union by painting a picture which had a basketball in the middle with a net in the upper right corner and a fist in the upper left corner. Upon completing this painting, she commented, "Ewing slamming." Ewing, then a very famous professional basketball for the New York Knicks, was Zana's basketball hero. A genuine integration of masculinity (the archetype of animus) into her feminine self appears to be taking place.

Sand picture 16

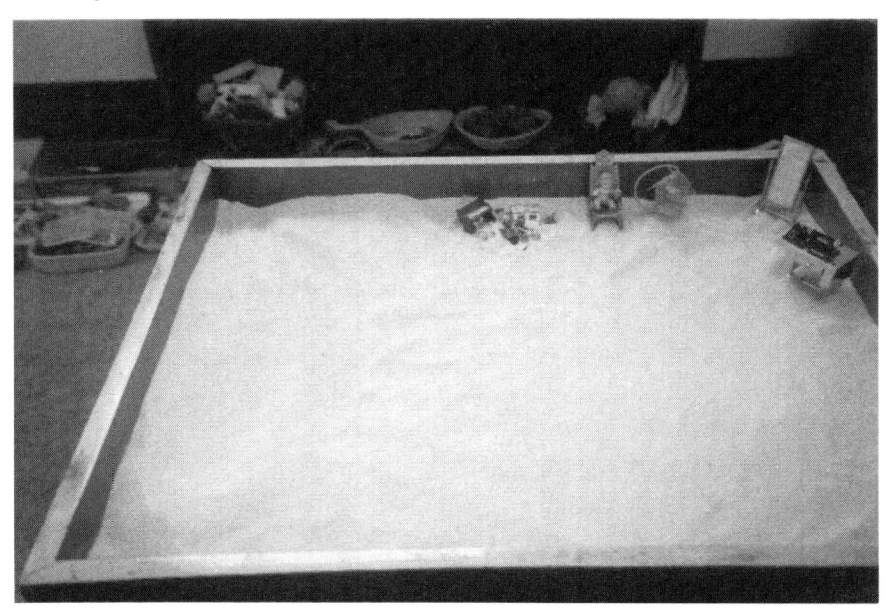

Figure 7.17 Baby on a golden throne.

Sand tray making process

In the beginning of this session, Zana and I planned a birthday party for her; her birthday was coming up the following week. She was very excited about this event. Then, she told me about a fight that she had had with a friend during basketball practice and shared with me her troublesome home condition. She had been temporarily staying with an aunt who, according to Zana, had been mean to her. She said her mother was out of town and she could not wait till her mother returned home in a few days. After sharing this information, Zana started a tray (Figure 7.17).

The first two items that she picked out were a golden throne and a baby. She proceeded to put the baby on the throne (upper middle). To the right of the baby was a bird's cage with a pink bird in it, whereas to the left of the baby, there was a treasure chest. Small toys around the chest were: five little figures (dolls); a key; a baby bottle; a large bottle; and a piano. In the upper right corner, there was a standing mirror and a sewing machine that had a telephone on top of it. In the left half of the tray, tracks were visible in the shape of a half-sun; they resembled sun rays that seemed to be shining.

Zana's comments

Upon completion of this tray, Zana said, "This is my friend's baby. She has a whole bunch of toys and has her own room. This baby is only eight or nine months old. She is real cute." She repeated, "This is my good friend's baby."

Therapist's interpretations

As noted by Esther Harding (1973, p. 167), the image of a child, possibly of a pregnancy and a birth, representing a rebirth of the personality, is likely to appear after a union of opposites appears in a tray. In Zana's case, following the theme of the union of the opposites in Figure 7.16, the birth of the baby is depicted here.

This baby is honored by sitting on a golden throne with a crown on top of the throne. The crown and the golden throne, normally belonging to a king, are known to be symbols of victory, honor and glory, and can also symbolize "spiritual enlightenment" (de Vries, 1984, p. 121). Together with the fact that we are planning to celebrate Zana's birthday, this baby seems a representation of her new birth. Moreover, its accompaniment by a standing mirror that is reflecting the shiny sun rays further depicts the bright future of this newborn baby.

The presence of a sewing machine that is capable of repairing defective materials and of creating new pieces of clothing represents a positive energy. The telephone that is sitting on top of the sewing machine suggests that in addition to the possession of new energy, there is a potential to communicate with the outer world.

Further strength is shown in the presence of the treasure chest with toys around it and the presence of a key. The key that can unlock the mystery and open the door to the future suggests that perhaps Zana is beginning to have the power of that key to unlock locked doors and solve her life mystery.

The presence of a bird in a cage seems to present a mixed message. As indicated by de Vries (1984, p. 75), the cage signifies man's contradictions (about marriage) because the birds outside long to get in, and those inside despair of getting out. It is likely that Zana, in her attempt to integrate the opposites, still has mixed feelings concerning this inner union. Overall, in spite of the frustration occurring in Zana's daily life, she seems to be on her way to a rebirth, albeit one that is still young and small—as depicted by all the very small items in this tray.

Subsequent to the making of this tray, in the next session, we celebrated Zana's birthday by having a party. She seemed very happy and shared a lot more information about herself. She did not make a tray on this day.

Sand picture 17

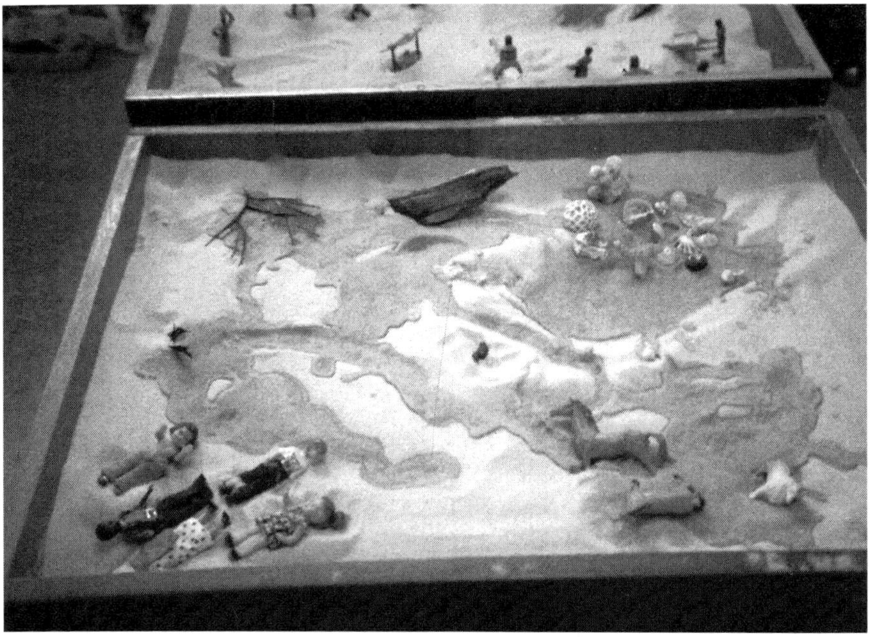

Figure 7.18 Total death.

After her birthday celebration, there was a session in which Zana painted another basketball picture (a game theme), made a clay work (a half-peeled banana, a baseball and a bat), and did a "partying" sand theme that was filled with animated figures, such as Dorothy with her traveling companions, the girl in a four-wheeler surrounded by Darth Vader, witches, gremlins, and a well-contained rainbow, sitting in the lower middle of the tray.

Around this time, Zana had been struggling with a tough decision (whether she would participate and reopen the court case against her perpetrator) because the perpetrator had recently committed intrusive acts on the family, i.e., stealing her mother's underwear and placing a composite picture of McDonald's, Zana, and her brother on their doorstep. The phallic clay work and the ambivalent party scene (Dorothy surrounded by good guys, and the girl in a four-wheeler surrounded by bad guys) seem to reflect her dilemma.

On this date, prior to her making this tray (Figure 7.18), Zana painted a picture of six balloons with the new paints I had brought in. She wrote, "Thanks" to indicate her appreciation. Since these balloons appear to go upwards, they fit Edinger's *sublimatio* symbolism (Edinger, 1985, p. 117). He noted, "*Sublimatio* is an ascent that raises us above the confining entanglements of immediate, earthy existence and its concrete, personal particulars. The higher we go, the grander and more comprehensive is our perspective" (p. 118). Perhaps Zana is attempting to fly higher in order to perceive her conflicted situation more objectively.

Sand tray making process

On this particular date, we chatted after playing two games of Uno. Zana talked mostly about the past and the ongoing family activities. Then she noticed the new paints which had been brought in and asked who brought them. After finding out that I had brought them in, she immediately painted a picture of balloons (please see the previous paragraph for details), using all new paint colors. Then she moved to the sand tray where she worked on the above scene (Figure 7.18) in a highly absorbed manner.

In the upper left corner, there was a coral fan. In the upper right quadrant, Zana placed many seashells, rocks, a starfish, and a small, lifeless swan. In between the coral fan and the pile of natural objects, there was dry driftwood. A limp blackbird lay in the middle of this tray. In between the dry driftwood and the blackbird, there was a piece of crystal. In the left middle of the tray, there were two little feathers. In the lower left quadrant, there were five figures—a grandmother figure, two boys, and two girls—all lying down motionless. In the lower right quadrant, there were two horses lying on their sides as well as a collie in the same position. In between the horses and the pile of natural objects, there was a chicken, also lifeless. Zana sprayed water over some parts of this tray.

Zana's comments

Zana said: "Everyone is cutting down the trees and the rainforest. They are killing animals. They are supposed to keep the green, but they do not. After they waste the nature, they will kill us, too."

Therapist's interpretations

There appears to be a very deep sense of anger, sadness, and despair portrayed in this highly destructive scene. The scene is a bit similar to the tray that she created two months ago (Figure 7.13), albeit a big difference is that the death or destruction in this tray is widespread and that nothing has survived. Although Zana did not verbally tell me much about her disturbing situation at home (her mother's job is threatened) and her extreme ambivalence about re-reporting the sexual abuse, she shared her deeply troublesome feelings through nonverbal means (this tray).

I was particularly struck by the water which was sprayed over the tray. It appeared to resemble tears, perhaps the tears that Zana shed over the sexual abuse and over losing her innocence, as well as for the inner anger and despair. However, the tears also remind me of Isis and Osiris. It was Isis's tears which brought together the fragments of Osiris's body and made them whole again (Edinger, 1985, p. 74). Moreover, both water and the crystal (located in between the dry driftwood and the blackbird) have a cleansing and purifying function. This may signify that Zana's further rebirth is on the way.

Sand picture 18

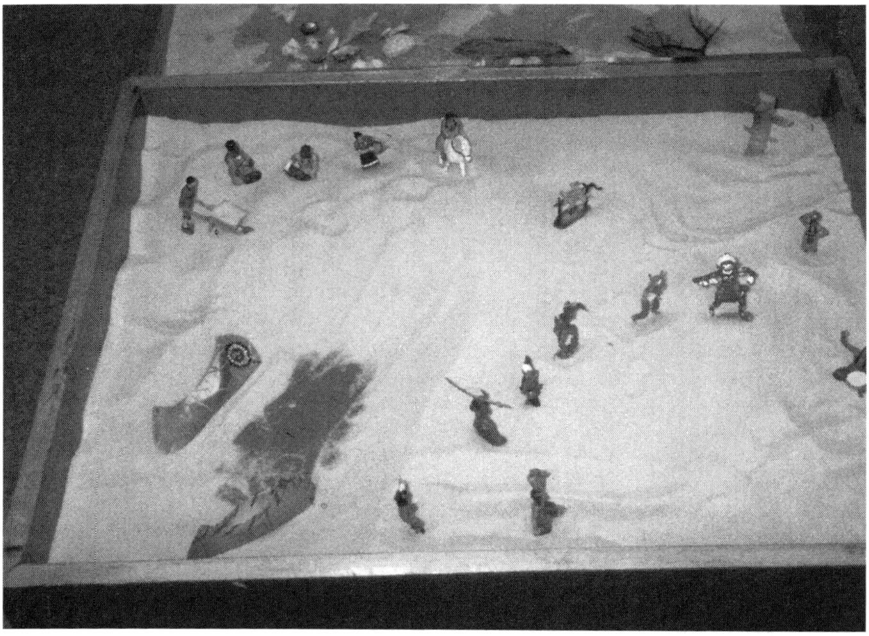

Figure 7.19a Execution.

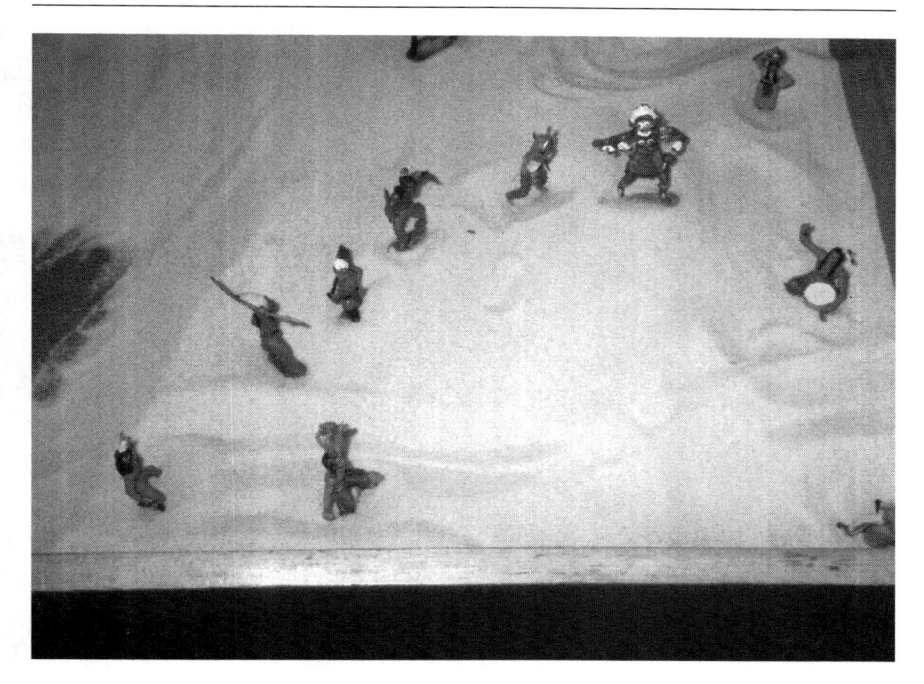

Figure 7.19b Execution detail (lower right corner).

Sand tray making process

Immediately after completing the destruction scene of Figure 7.18, Zana went to work on the dry tray (Figure 7.19a). In the upper left quadrant, five Native American women were working; they were pushing a wheelbarrow, mixing food, carrying a papoose, carrying food, and riding a horse. In the lower left quadrant, two canoes were resting by the lake. In the lower right quadrant, there was a group of eight Native American males, including two medicine men; they carried either weapons or drums. In the lowest right corner (Figure 7.19b), a Native American male was tied to a post that had a hatchet and a skull on top of it (only partially seen). In the middle right, a Native American female was standing by, facing the lower right males. A fire roasting a beast was put in the middle of the tray. In the upper right corner, a totem pole was placed.

Zana's comments

At completion, Zana briefly remarked: "Back when Indians were here, there was no white man."

Therapist's interpretations

After the making of a very destructive scene, a beautiful and what seems to be a peaceful ceremonial scene appears. However, on closer inspection, I see a scene of execution taking place in the latter tray. This theme was somewhat puzzling to me. Much later, I learned that Zana's perpetrator is a middle-aged, Native American male. I began to wonder if perhaps Zana, on an unconscious level, was performing an execution ritual of the perpetrator in this sand tray.

The woman (right middle) standing by observing the execution scene perhaps represents Zana's strengthening observing ego, capable of helping her to work through this ordeal. The fire and the roasting food, two boats which can transport people and goods, and a protective totem pole signify warmth, nurturing, communication, and protection. Psychologically speaking and symbolically, Zana has nailed the perpetrator to the cross, has liberated herself from the shame associated with the victimization, and she has triumphed.

On this particular day, all four essential elements are present: earth (represented by sand); air (represented by the flying balloons); fire (the fire that is used for roasting); and water (the small lake with two boats nearby). This may represent her return to *prima materia*, or what Edinger (1985, p. 11) calls the formless state of pure potentiality in order to facilitate further transformation. Indeed, a genuine transformation appears to have taken place.

Sand picture 19

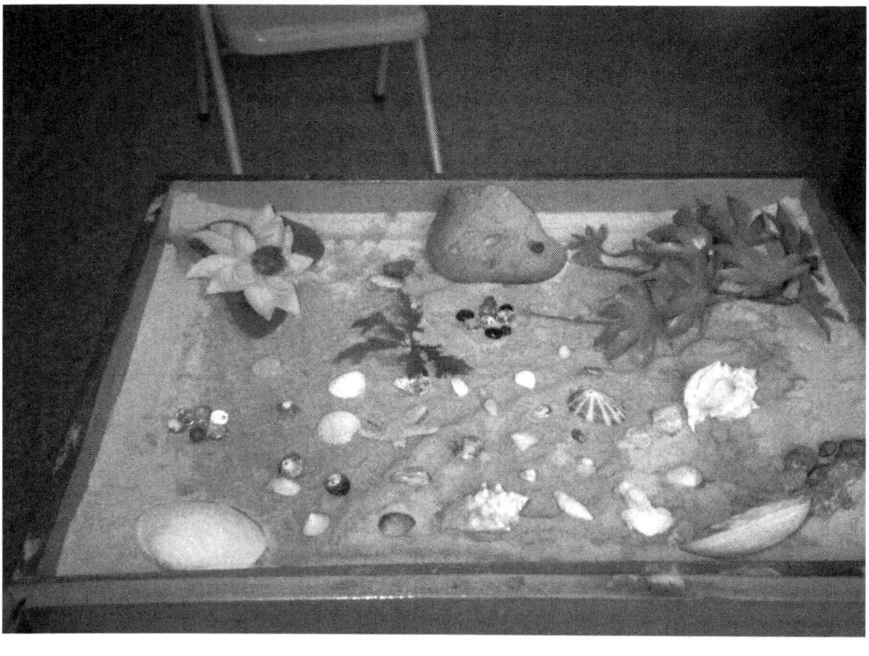

Figure 7.20 Bottom of the ocean.

Sand tray making process

In the beginning of the session, Zana and I planned a party for the last session, which was scheduled two weeks from this date. She volunteered to bring brownies, cookies, and balloons. Then we had a brief discussion concerning her position about reopening the sexual abuse case. She decided against reopening the case because she could not recall the details any longer. She indicated that she was comfortable with this decision. Then, she went immediately to the tray and made this beautiful bottom-of-the-ocean scene (Figure 7.20).

She spread many shells and rocks of different sizes and shapes all over this tray. Two small piles of glass marbles were placed in the middle left and near the upper middle. Two tree branches, one red (in the near middle) and one green (in the upper right corner) were present. In the upper middle, there was a large rock formation. In the upper left corner, a large lotus flower bloomed. Zana poured water all over the tray.

Zana's comments

Upon completion, Zana stated briefly: "This is what the bottom of the ocean looks like."

Therapist's interpretations

I truly believe that this beautiful bottom-of-the-ocean scene represents the manifestation of the Self as described by Kalff. The union of the masculine and the feminine aspects is harmoniously presented by the balanced rock formation and by the evenly distributed and gorgeously displayed shells. Two piles of multicolored glass marbles which are in a mandala shape seem to reflect the light of the inner self. Moreover, the colorful tree branches appear full of life.

The most impressive aspect of this tray is the presence of a huge, beautiful lotus arising out of the bottom of the ocean. The lotus is known to be both solar and lunar, representing both spirit and matter, and is associated with renaissance, creation, fecundity, renewal, immortality, and the perfection of beauty (Cooper, 1979, p. 100).

In Chinese, the lotus is the symbol of purity and perfection because it grows out of mud, but is not defiled—just as Buddha is born into the world, but lives above it—and because its fruits are said to be ripe when the flower blooms—just as the truth preached by Buddha immediately bears the fruit of enlightenment (Williams, 1976, p. 257). In addition, every part of the lotus has a name and is useful to the Chinese (Williams, 1976, p. 256).

A genuine transformation has taken place; Zana has arisen out of the mud (having been sexually abused in the past), purified and transformed.

Moreover, a reconciliation and union of her inner masculinity and femininity has occurred. She appears ready to shine her light as depicted by the colorful marbles in the mandala-like circles and to be useful in the future.

On this same date, after making the sand tray, Zana made two pictures and a sticker design. A picture of four flowers was made, following her "Rain and snow go away!" picture. Zana entitled this picture, "April showers bring May flowers." These four flowers seem to amplify the lotus that she had placed in the sand tray. Number four is known as a symbol of wholeness (Jung, 1968, p. 234) and suggests that Zana has finally reached the aim of her journey—finding inner wholeness.

Sand picture 20

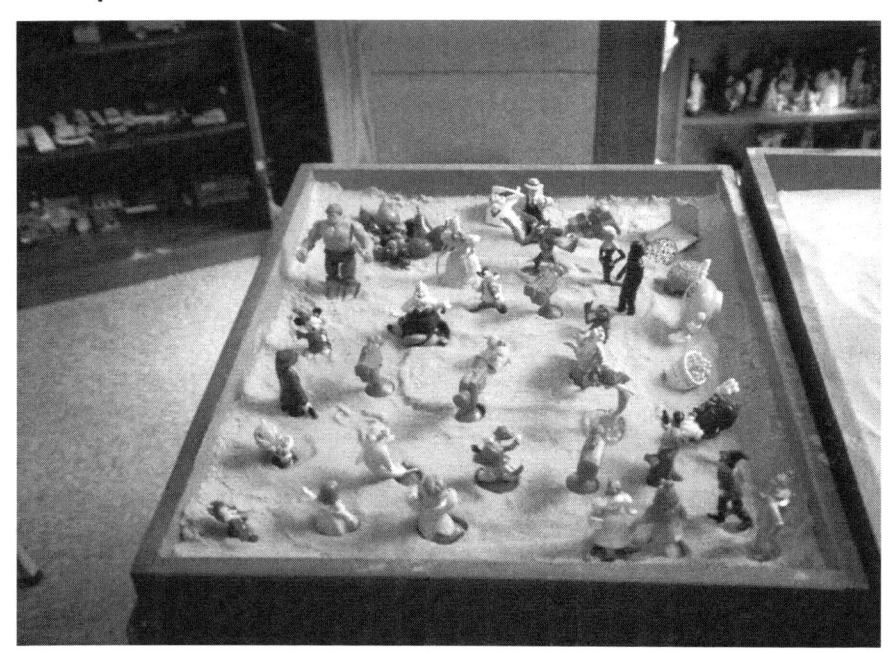

Figure 7.21 A lively party.

Sand tray making process

On this date, Zana and I had another brief discussion about the party for the last session and her feelings about not testifying against her perpetrator. Zana felt fine about her decision not to testify, and she felt safe. She asked me a few personal questions. Then she began to work on the sand tray (Figure 7.21). Similar to most sand trays that she had made, she was very absorbed in this task.

Lots of food, including many kinds of fruits, pizza, and the food from McDonald's were present in the upper quadrant, mainly in the outskirt area.

Characters from various fairy tales, movies, and shows were spread all over the tray, including Dorothy and all her friends from *The Wizard of Oz* (the lower right corner). All the characters formed a circle with Yoda standing right in the middle. Four (pink) cameras were placed among the characters.

Zana's comments

Zana titled this tray: "What if TV characters came to life?"

Therapist's interpretions

This is clearly a lively celebration scene. All of the characters seem to be participating in some sort of action, either marching in a parade or dancing. In addition, there seems to be a circling action. Yoda is now surrounded by friendly figures and is in the center of this tray. The balance of male and female figures suggests an integration of inner masculinity and femininity. The availability of abundant food, especially the pizza which is no longer contained in a box, indicates the presence of ready and plentiful resources. Four cameras, in contrast to the one camera in Figure 7.1, are available to film this festive party. Overall, this is a lively party or, psychologically, a celebration of a new life for Zana.

Sand picture 21

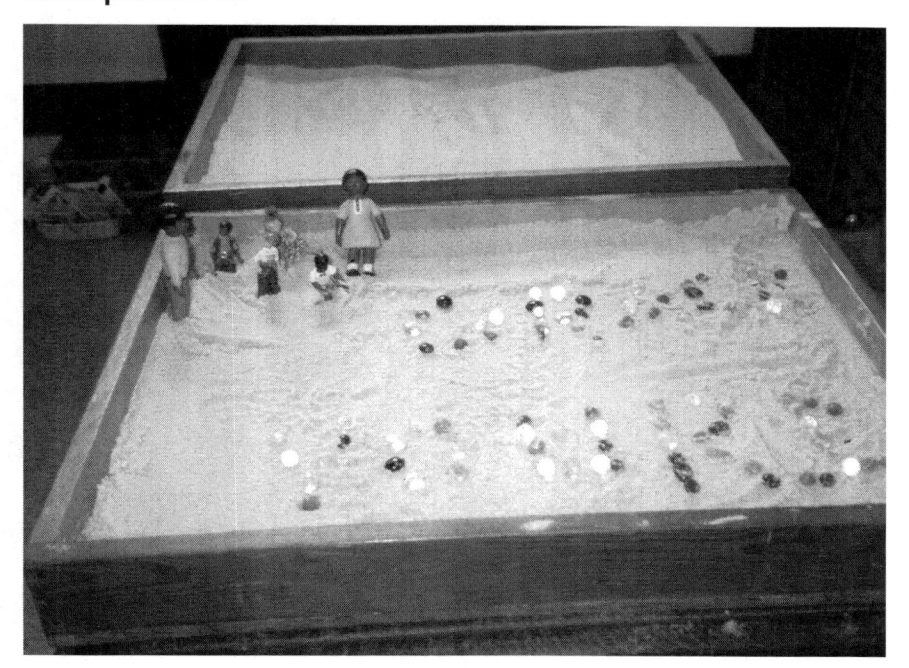

Figure 7.22 Goodbye and thanks.

Sand tray making process

During this last session, Zana and I held a party. We shared the food we brought, and then we had a review of all the pictures that she had made. Zana carefully wrote down what I told her about the pictures. Then she asked to make another tray. While making this tray, she commented that while she didn't know how many children I had seen for the therapy project, she decided to put six children in the tray.

In this tray (Figure 7.22), she arranged colorful glass marbles to spell, "GRACE YOUR 1." Then, she placed six children, including the black girl in the yellow dress, in the upper left corner.

Zana's comments

Upon completion of this tray, Zana and I stood in front of the tray and marveled at it for a moment; neither Zana nor I said a word.

Therapist's interpretations

There was no need for Zana to say anything. The tray speaks for itself. Grace is my first name, and Zana put it in the tray to say "You are number one in my heart." This act represents her appreciation for all the work that she and I had done together. Since the marbles she uses in this tray are also present in the tray that she labeled "My journey" (Figure 7.11) and the Self tray of "The bottom of the ocean" (Figure 7.20), I wonder if Zana is carrying the light we shared together in this process with her for her future life journey.

Chapter 8

Summary

Zana is an 11½-year-old Caucasian female. She was one of the ten subjects chosen by the school social worker for a sandplay therapy outcome study. One of the main criteria used for choosing the subjects was their need for therapy.

Zana was the victim of repeated sexual abuse by a neighbor, a Native American and part-African American male, during the summer when she was 8 years old. The abuse included intercourse and penetration by numerous objects. Even though Zana and her family reported the offense to the police, a miscommunication between the Child Protection Agency and the police resulted in the perpetrator not being prosecuted, unfortunately. He still lived in Zana's neighborhood at the time of this sandplay process.

At the intake, Zana was observed to be quite passive, reserved, sad, and nonverbal, but also friendly and cooperative. The Children's Depression Inventory, an instrument used for initial assessment, suggested that Zana was severely depressed (the score was twenty-four). Upon completion of therapy, Zana's Children's Depression Inventory Index score was within normal limits. In addition, her projective drawings suggested that she was "more confident, less anxious, and less confused."

At the post-therapy testing, her Rorschach protocol indicated that she was happier, not as distressed, and that she had better reality perception. Two evaluators blindly interpreted the pre- and post-therapy projective drawings as well as the Rorschach protocols. They did not know which set was pre or post. They were able to accurately pick out the post-therapy protocols. This implies that Zana's emotional functioning had significantly improved, thus the evaluators could discern the improvement based on blind interpretations.

Throughout the entire process, regardless of what she did, Zana appeared to try her best and to make the most of her time. In twenty sessions, she produced a total of twenty-four sand pictures; eight paint, crayon, or chalk pictures; four sticker art designs; and four clay sculptures.

At the outset (Figure 7.1, "The initial searching"), Zana spelled out her inner barrenness, her ego–Self alienation, her need for protection, and her goal of searching for inner wholeness and spiritual rebirth. She also indicated a desire to integrate her inner splits, including a need to resolve racial and sexual issues. In the second sand picture (Figure 7.2, "Down to the shadowy land") she made, also during her first session, she descended into the dark unconsciousness realm. This sand tray clearly depicted her severe depression; her desire to confront the shadow, including the sexual victimization; and her yearning for a rebirth of her psyche.

The two trays that she made during the second session (Figure 7.3, "Grandmother is visiting!" and Figure 7.4, "Animals are out") again reflected her alienated ego, her depression, and her need for transformation. The beginning of a co-transference was evident when she shared some emotional information with me during the second session. By the third session, it appeared that I had passed the transference test. It is commonly known in the sandplay community that a therapist must pass the transference test in order for the client to make significant progress. In this session, Zana eagerly shared her crisis situation—the perceived mistreatment she had received from her basketball coach. As she was sharing, she painted a picture (Figure 7.5, "Peace?"). Together, we worked out a coping strategy.

During the fifth session (Figure 7.7, "Children, Santa Claus, and animals"), a genuine transformation at her ego–Self axis seemed to have taken place. Santa Claus was used as a bridge symbol, which brought integration of love versus fear and of conscious versus unconscious.

The first manifestation of Self represented by the drawing of a big circle occurred right after the placing of a bridge symbol (Figure 7.7 and Figure 7.8, "Black as a president?"). In addition, Zana seemed to move from what Kalff coined the animal-vegetative stage into a fighting stage.

After her willingness to show inner barrenness as manifested in Figure 7.9, "My room," Zana became ready to take on the world, as represented by the Dorothy figure standing on a huge mound in Figure 7.10, "On top of the world." Dorothy, a white figure, also seemed to reflect Zana's ready acceptance of being a Caucasian girl among the majority of black and Native Americans in her school. In order to brave the world, Zana made a large number of food items (clay works), the nourishment for her soul journey.

In the eighth session (Figure 7.11, "My journey"), Zana made a tray that depicted self-assertiveness and determination; she indicated that this sand picture represented her journey and that she could make her own decisions. The light of her life appeared to be shining through the glass marbles that she placed in this picture. As she journeyed on, she ran into a "demon" (Figure 7.12, "The demon"). An attempt on her part to integrate the opposites was beautifully represented by the story she shared about the dragon in this picture.

In the next few trays (Figure 7.13, "The destruction," Figure 7.14, "The wedding," and Figure 7.15, "Save the school"), Zana appeared to be struggling a great deal with the union of opposites. In addition, she appeared to be attempting to integrate the archetypal animus into her psyche.

By the thirteenth session (Figure 7.16, "They are marrying"), a giant step towards the union of opposites seemed to have taken place. The basketball player and the bride in this sand tray were truly getting married. Integration or the union of the active masculine principle and the passive feminine principle was clearly depicted in this picture. Subsequent to this union, a new Self was born as represented by the baby sitting on a golden throne with a crown on top of it and the reflection of shiny sun rays (Figure 7.17, "Baby on a golden throne").

When Zana turned 12, a crisis appeared. The perpetrator of the sexual abuse was suspected of entering the house, taking and leaving items; the need for her to re-report the offense was brought up. Her anxiety and ambivalence concerning the matter were projected onto some sand pictures. In particular, the "Total death" scene in Figure 7.18 reflected her inner despair and anguish. On the same date, in the second tray (Figure 7.19) that she made, an "Execution" scene was enacted. Symbolically, she nailed her perpetrator to a cross and executed him.

Following that session, she became very comfortable about not re-reporting the offense. In the next sand picture (Figure 7.20, "Bottom of the ocean"), a genuinely beautiful manifestation of the Self was evident. The presence of a beautiful lotus blossom arising out of the ocean seemed to represent her new self, the one which was capable of rising above all difficulties.

Zana ended her sandplay process by creating a scene of celebration for her new life (Figure 7.21, "A lively party"), and a "Goodbye and thanks" scene in Figure 7.22. At this time, we both knew that the work or the *opus* was completed. However, we both realized that this was just a new beginning and that there would be further work in the future.

In a subsequent follow-up two years later, I learned that Zana had adjusted well in a new charter school, where she served as vice-president on the student council. She had grown many inches in height, and had become a physically mature young lady. She was very pleased to see me and eager to share new information.

In a retrospective manner, she summarized the benefits of the sandplay therapy to her in the following four areas. First of all, she felt she had better coping skills. In this regard, she explained that when things went wrong, she knew how to express her feelings and how to be more assertive in order to solve her problems. Second, she felt that she had better self-confidence. Third, she realized that she could look at things more objectively. Lastly, she had better self-reflection.

When questioned about the sexual abuse, Zana indicated that she did not think about it any more and that she felt safe. She added that sometimes she saw the perpetrator in the neighborhood and felt sorry for him because he looked old and frail.

In regards to her family life, she stated that she got along well with her family members, especially her brother, who was the president of the student council at the same school. In addition, both her brother and her mother were on the school board. At this point, her father was still living at home, gravely ill. Zana commented that although she had mixed feelings about his dying, she felt it would be all right with her if he chose to leave the world. She was very sympathetic about his suffering.

All in all, Zana seemed to have adjusted rather well since we parted about two years ago. Most importantly, it was such a great privilege for me to work with Zana, and the experience truly was one of the most rewarding ones that I have had, especially knowing that Zana had genuinely transformed through the process.

Part III

Study of the symbol

Chapter 9

Importance of symbol in sandplay therapy

The symbol occupies an important role in sandplay therapy; to study and to know symbols is essential in sandplay therapy training and practice. The symbols represent a bridge, or a means that help us enter into a client's inner world. As Katherine Bradway pointed out, the nonverbal sandplay approach will bring clients back to an early developmental stage in which visual images, not verbal words, are main tools of communication (Bradway and McCoard, 2005, p. 89). Because of sandplay's ability to relate to events that occurred in the preverbal stage, it can also be used to heal the deep-seated trauma that happened in the same stage.

To qualify as a competent sandplay therapist, one must study and understand symbols. In order to be certified as a clinical member of the International Society of Sandplay Therapy or Sandplay Therapists of America, a therapist must write a symbol paper that meets the ISST's or the STA's standards of the association. In an article that Barbara Weller wrote, entitled "So you have to write a symbol paper!", Weller clearly spelled out that in order to really understand and to write about a symbol, one must relate it to one's personal experience; know its objective data; learn about its meaning in traditional religions, mythological creation stories, and fairy tales; and know its meanings as commonly understood in Jungian analytical theories.

Responding to Weller's article, Pratibha Eastwood (1999) further illustrated that there are three stages in studying a symbol: Impetus; Leela, the Divine Dance; and Finding Form. During the Impetus stage, one begins to choose a symbol to study. It can be mysterious, unexplainable; one may be irrationally attracted to this symbol. This symbol may present in one's dreams or in one's sand trays. Following such a stage, one enters the Leela, the Divine Dance stage. This stage may be characterized by free-flowing exploration; it is like a divine dance that is playful, automatic, perhaps confusing, and yet, very joyful and exciting. In the last stage of Finding Form, the object of the study, the symbol, will become organized and integrated. It will be related to archetypal images, will be represented in real forms, and its researcher will finally realize why he or she chose this symbol to study and how it plays in his or her inner transformation.

In Chapter 10, I will present my own symbol study story in which there is the initial confusion and struggling, the exciting exploration, and the eventual integration. In researching my symbol, the dragon, I encountered many challenges, surprises, and joy. My symbol study is a research paper that meets the ISST and STA certification requirement standards. I am proud to point out that during the research process, I became an artist; I painted a dragon picture that hangs on my living-room wall.

Chapter 10

Study of the dragon as a symbol

Introduction

I would like to start with a story about a man whose marriage was in trouble, as was told in Anthony de Mello's *One Minute Wisdom* (1985, p. 175). The man sought a master's advice, and the master said, "You must learn to listen to your wife." The man went home and took his master's advice to heart. He returned after a month and told the master that he had learned to listen to every word his wife said. The master smiled and said, "Now go home and listen to every word she isn't saying."

The study of the dragon has been an extremely difficult and challenging task for me. There were times when I felt totally confused by it, and there were times when I felt enlightened. I will try to present the dragon to you in the best possible way, and yet I know that I will leave out important parts which may or may not need to be known. Therefore, I would like to invite you to listen to every word that I say and also to every word that I don't say.

First of all, I would like to share my struggle with picking out the dragon as my symbol. Initially, I chose the horse for my symbol study simply because I was born in the Year of the Horse, according to the Chinese zodiac. The Chinese zodiac has a twelve-year cycle; a different animal or affinity symbolizes each year. The horse corresponds with the seventh year of the cycle, two years after the Year of the Dragon. When the study of symbol was initiated, I instinctively chose the symbol of the horse. However, I grew uncomfortable with this decision though I could not discern exactly why. Consequently, I began to search for a different symbol. Suddenly, the symbol of the dragon entered my mind.

I remembered that, as a child the dragon greatly fascinated me, partly because my older brother, the first-born son of the family, was born under the Year of the Dragon. I idolized my brother in our childhood because he excelled at everything. Not only did he get the best grades, but also he was the fastest runner in the whole school. When both he and I were nominated as candidates for student council president, I campaigned more eagerly for him than I did for myself. I envied him and his affinity—the dragon. I distinctly remembered that my mother had commented on how she registered my brother as being born under the Year of the Dragon rather than the Year of the Snake (the following year) simply because he was born at twilight of December 31 and January 1 and because the dragon symbolized good luck. I should add that even though it is commonly known that the Chinese affinity goes with the lunar calendar, in Taiwan most people use the solar calendar as a reference for affinity. My mother certainly did that when she made that comment.

In Taiwan, my native country, many parents like to have sons born in the Year of the Dragon, not only because it symbolizes good luck, but also because it is the symbol of the king. There is a Chinese saying, "Wang-Zu-Tseng-Long," which literally means, "Wishing children to become dragons." This phrase reflects parents' aspirations for their children to become successful and famous.

As a child, I was drawn to many dragon stories, especially those that pertained to the daughter of the dragon king of the sea. These stories were usually about the love that developed between a human being—most often a poor and kind young man—and the daughter of the dragon king of the sea. The magic powers, the beauty of the daughter, the wonderful palace in which the sea dragon king resided, and the treasures, were all intriguing, fascinating, and also a bit frightening to me. Adults would sometimes scold their children when they were misbehaving by saying, "Why don't you marry the daughter of the dragon king of the sea?", meaning, "Why don't you just get out of my face?" Because I could not recall the details of the stories of the dragon king's daughter, I requested the help of a knowledgeable friend. This friend sent me the following short story.

> Ashiao, a very poor fisherman, lived with his elderly mother; he relied on his daily fishing to support her. Every time he caught any fish, he sold them to a very rich man who owned many acres of land. People called the rich man the Lord of the Ten Thousand Acres. One day, Ashiao caught an extremely beautiful carp, but did not sell it to the lord because he wanted to give it to his mother as a birthday gift. Upon seeing such a beautiful carp, Ashiao's mother was very pleased. When she began to scale the fish, she saw tears coming out of its eyes. She was astonished and decided to release the fish back to the sea.
>
> Ashiao returned to the seashore with the intention of letting the fish go. The Lord of the Ten Thousand Acres, who was looking to buy some fish from Ashiao, was there. When the lord saw the majestic fish, he demanded that Ashiao give it to him. Out of loyalty to his mother, Ashiao refused to sell the fish to the lord. As the two men struggled, Ashiao threw the fish back into the sea. The lord grew incensed and swore that he would not buy any more fish from Ashiao.
>
> One day, while Ashiao was fishing, a beautiful young lady suddenly

appeared behind him. She sat upon the seashore to watch him fish. They fell in love at first sight, and Ashiao took her home to marry her. Ashiao's mother was ecstatic that Ashiao had married such a beautiful and obedient wife. Since the wife's arrival at Ashiao's house, the family grew in love and in wealth.

Soon, the Lord of the Ten Thousand Acres noticed that Ashiao had grown richer and had a beautiful wife. The lord vowed to have revenge on Ashiao. Since the lord had great power, he manipulated the government to commit Ashiao to prison on the charges of kidnapping a young lady (Ashiao's wife). When Ashiao's mother learned that her son had been detained by the police, she wept bitter tears. She wanted to rescue her son. The lord sent Ashiao's mother a messenger who informed her that if she would send Ashiao's wife to the lord, the lord would send one of his wives to Ashiao, plus half of his land. Ashiao's mother agreed to the deal. As soon as the deal was signed, Ashiao was released from jail. The lord had a celebration upon obtaining the most beautiful wife in the land. He had a pagoda built on the seashore, and he wanted to have a dragon boat race as part of the celebration. The lord and his new wife were on one of the dragon boats, and the lord had his wife in a tight embrace. The wife suddenly fell into the sea, dragging the lord along with her. That was the end of the Lord of the Ten Thousand Acres.

It was commonly thought that Ashiao's beautiful wife was the daughter of the dragon king of the sea and also was the beautiful carp that was transformed. Therefore, when the Lord of the Ten Thousand Acres fell into the sea, people saw a carp jumping out of the water before going back into the sea. Most people believe that the carp had returned to her father, the dragon king of the sea.

This story hit home. Some of my repressed memories came alive. Not only did I wish that I had been born in the Year of the Dragon, but also I wished that I had been the daughter of the dragon king of the sea—beautiful, magical, adored, loved, and away from human troubles. Those were my wishes whenever I encountered problems during my childhood.

When I decided to make the dragon the symbol of my study, I instantly relaxed. Around that time, I came across a passage in Francis Huxley's book, *The dragon* (1979), which contained a Japanese aphorism that stated, "In heaven a horse is made into a dragon, among men, a dragon is made into a horse" (Huxley, 1992, p. 20). Huxley pointed out that the Japanese sacrificed horses at the spring festival and when the gods withheld the rain. The horses were sent to heaven, where they became dragons. There, they presided over the change of water into fire and fire back into water. This connection between the horse and the dragon truly astonished me.

I knew that I could not merely dismiss it as a coincidence. It felt to me as if it was what Jung called synchronicity. When I looked at pictures of my sandplay process, I noticed that while horses appeared in the earlier trays, a dragon appeared in the final tray. I did my sandplay process before I had ever read Francis Huxley's aphorism, so this was another amazing example of synchronicity. Moreover, I had pasted a card with several horses on it and a card with several dragons on it to the inside cover of a special box which I had made for my attachment work. The horse card was on the top and the dragon card was on the bottom. Again, I made this special box several months before I had chosen the dragon for my symbol study. Perhaps horses could be transformed into dragons and my childhood wishes could come true? Of interest and perhaps significantly, on the day I decided to study the symbol of the dragon, two of the four clients in my research project incorporated the dragon in their sand trays. One of the two who had a dragon in her tray was Zana. Please see Figure 7.12 for details.

Did the dragon ever exist?

In earliest Chinese mythology, the dragon represented the dynasties. For example, the first and second dynasties of mythology were documented as the Nine-Dragon Dynasty and the Five-Dragon Dynasty respectively. A number of the earliest famous Chinese kings were associated with the dragon. The kings were either born to a dragon ancestry or they appeared in the form of dragons themselves. Many Chinese people believed that dragons did exist, once upon a time; Chinese people considered the dragon noble and perhaps sacred. In contrast, Western society had more doubts as to the existence of dragons.

In their book, *The book of the dragon*, Judy Allen and Jeanne Griffiths (1979) indicated that even though the dragon as a symbol has been used in most cultures throughout the history of the world, they do not think that dragons exist. On the other hand, in *Dragons and unicorns*, Paul and Karin Johnsgard (1982) noted that doubting the existence of dragons is due to people's limited intelligence and closed minds (1982). In *The flight of dragons*, Peter Dickinson (1979) suggested that there are three views concerning the existence of these glorious animals. First, they are completely legendary. Second, they are largely legendary, but contain elements based on second-hand accounts of real animals—crocodiles, boa constrictors, sting rays, and so on. Third, they really exist. Dickinson (1979) indicated that he believed in the third view.

Because I was brought up in Asia, I tend to believe that the dragon may have existed in the earlier history of the world, perhaps right around creation time. The dragon has played a big role in my life, especially in my childhood fantasies and presumed realities. At this point, I somehow feel that my life perhaps has been and will be guided, to some extent, by this symbol as well as by the symbol of the horse. That is my affinity in the Chinese zodiac. Psychologically and symbolically speaking, I deem the integration of the dragon and the horse or the transformation from a horse into a dragon or into the daughter of the dragon king of the sea to be one of my important life tasks.

Dragons in mythology, folklore, and religion

The authors of *The book of the dragon* (Allen and Griffiths, 1979) indicated that according to the *Encyclopedia Britannica*, the word dragon was derived through the French and Latin from the Greek *drakon*, connected with *derkomai*, "sea," and interpreted as sharp-sighted. Furthermore, they said that the equivalent English word "drake" or "fire-drake" was derived from the Anglo-Saxon *draca*. They stated that in Greece, the word *drakon* was originally used to denote any large serpent, and the dragon of mythology, whatever the shape it may have assumed, remains essentially a snake. Thus, they pointed out that dragon and serpent mythology were closely interwoven.

In the Book of Revelation in the Holy Bible (Chapter 12, Verse 9), there is a reference to the great dragon as the old snake or the serpent from the book of Genesis (Chapter 3, Verse 1). It, the great dragon, was regarded as the devil who deceived the world. Most people who have read the Bible know that the serpent skillfully and strategically led Eve and Adam to disobey God. This, I think, has contributed to the Western view of the dragon as a destructive force.

Allen and Griffiths (1979) also stated that the major symbolic roles of the serpent/dragon were: the creator of most ancient manifestations of the emerging spirit; the chaos which had to be overcome for the world to be properly ordered; the encircler of the earth or the monster who kept back the waters; the spirit or guardian of the earth or underworld; the cosmic enemy, the amorphous, serpent-dragon who personifies the powers of darkness and has to be overcome at dawn and at sunset; the fertility spirit—chiefly in the form of the corn-god; the water-god, especially living in the caverns out of which the Nile flood was believed to have come; the distinguished form of the non-human—the serpent is a primeval creature living in the dark earth or the depth of the water, uncanny and hostile, and possibly very wise. Allen and Griffiths (1979) further pointed out that both the dragon and the serpent are connected with immortality, having to do with their ability to shed their skins and emerge slightly larger and brighter than before.

Here is another source of the dragon symbol that Allen and Griffths (1979) provided. In Mexico, the origin of the plumed serpent was known as Quetzalcoatl. Quetzal was a rare bird with green feathers and inhabited the highlands of Chipas and Guatemala. It lived in the tops of trees and was distinguishable from other birds because it had two front toes and very small claws. Coatl was also the Nahua word for snake, but combined *co*, a generic name for serpent in the Mayan language, and *atl*, the Nahuan word for water. Therefore, Quetzalcoatl was the Mexican equivalent of the Mayan Kukulcan which represented the divine, the serpent, the number four, and the feathered.

The dragon, or the feathered serpent of South America and Mexico, appeared to be central to the mythology of the countries' respective religions. It was associated with power, fertility, weather phenomena, the life force, and resurrection.

The dragon was known to be "the seductress in the waters": Huxley (1992, p. 72) noted that the dragon's daughters are famed for their beauty, their wisdom, their singing and their dancing, and other erotic accomplishments. Huxley also pointed out that the dragon was the weather-maker. He noted that the dragon of the Caribbean is believed to be responsible for earthquakes (p. 74)

Similarly, in Chinese mythology, the Shen Lung was known to be the mightiest in power of the eight orders of the Chinese dragonhood (Baskin and Baskin, 1985). Baskin and Baskin (1985) noted that Shen Lung's realm of control was very extensive, including the sky, the ocean, and the earth. Because of his enormous power, Shen Lung would become tired and lazy; he chose to disguise himself as a mouse, hiding in either a house or in the woods. The thunder god, in need of Shen Lung's work, would send servants all over to look for him. When Shen Lung was found, the thunder god would punish him by striking. That is why in a thunderstorm, there is thunder and lightning around the woods and the top of houses. Shun Lung was also the one who showed up in the Chinese New Year parade celebration. His outer appearance would be very colorful, shimmering and shining; he would vibrate and quiver in a trembling rainbow of brilliant colors as he moved along (Baskin and Baskin, 1985, p. 13).

The contrast between Eastern and Western dragons

In the book, *St. George and the dragon* (1984), as retold by Margaret Hodges, the following descriptions depicted the terrible dragon:

> Then they heard a hideous roaring that filled the air with terror and seemed to shake the ground. The dreadful dragon lay stretched on the sunny side of a great hill, like a great hill himself, and when he saw the knight's armor glistening in the sunlight, he came eagerly to do battle . . . His great size made a wide shadow under his huge body as a mountain casts a shadow on a valley. He reared high, monstrous, horrible and vast, armed all over with scales of brass fitted so closely that no sword or spear can pierce them . . . A cloud of smothering smoke and burning sulfur poured from his throat, filling the air with its stench. His blazing eyes, flaming with rage, glared out from deep within his head. So raising his speckled breast, the dragon rushed towards the knight, clashing his scales, as he leapt to greet his newest victim.

In contrast, Williams (1976, p. 132) stated the following about the dragon:

"The Eastern dragon is not the gruesome monster of medieval imagination, but the genius of strength and goodness. He is the spirit of change, therefore of life itself."

McGowen (1981) noted that the

> Chinese dragons were highly civilized and had their own kingdom with a government and laws. And unlike the troublesome European dragons, Chinese dragons were generally kind and helpful to humans. They often appeared in human forms, usually as a man with a large mouth, a green beard, and dragon horns sprouting from his head.

In the book, *The truth about dragons*, Blumberg (1980) indicated, "A few dragons begin life as fish." Carp that successfully jump up and leap over waterfalls change into fish-dragons.

A popular Chinese phrase *li-yu tiao lung-mung* (The carp has leapt through the dragon's gate) means success, for example students who have passed the exams or graduated. I would like to interject that near the completion of my doctoral degree program, I received a precious present from a relative—it was a dress with a design of a carp leaping through a gate. This gift represented this relative's wish for me to successfully complete the program and to be successful in my profession.

Comparisons of Eastern and Western dragons were made in this and previous sections: here is a summary. In Eastern Asia, the following images of the dragon are predominant: benevolent; beautiful; friendly; wise; genius of strength and goodness; spirit of change; powerful and transforming; angelic; loving; reverent; anything associated with the king. In the Western world, the images associated with the dragon are quite gloomy. They might include: evil; destructive; ugly; nasty; mean; gruesome; terrible; terrifying; monstrous; dangerous; disgusting. The Western dragons are also known to spread diseases and plagues, to have poison tanks, and to be murderous.

Slaying the dragon

Allen and Griffiths (1979) wrote an interesting chapter on slaying the dragon (pp. 118–126). As they noted, the slaying of the dragon was largely a Western phenomenon. In the Far East, the dragon was never slain and could not be slain because the dragon was a vision, a light in the sky, and an apparition in the water. In Western literature, the dragon was put to the sword or other forms of slaying for one reason or another, including the darkness, the evil, and the chaos that needed to be conquered.

According to Allen and Griffiths (1979), the importance of the slaying depended upon what the dragon was seen to represent. Some of the representations of the dragon include: The Primal Waters; the darkness—the dark and unconscious side of humankind; the force of evil or the devil himself; the devourer; the thief of immortality; the alchemical symbol of *prima materia*; the guardian of the hoard. The important emphasis for these researchers is that, while the dragon transmutes and changes, it is not destroyed—the original elements are still contained within.

The same authors pointed out:

> In essence, the symbols of immortality were there: the incorruptible gold, associated with the sun which set only to rise again; the lunar pearl (guarded by the dragon), associated with the moon which waned and waxed full again; and the serpent are symbols of death and resurrection. Therefore, the dragon held immortality. (Allen and Griffiths, 1979, p. 66)

This echoed the old alchemical text that stated "The dragon slays itself, weds itself, impregnates itself," in a philosophical cycle of "exist, destroy, create" (Allen and Griffiths, 1979, p. 66).

Psychologically, Jung depicted the dragon as representing the initial stage of the unconscious; he believed that the unconscious must be sacrificed in order to enter the realm of conscious knowledge and understanding (Allen and Griffiths, 1979).

As for me, in this life, the dragon seems to represent the pure gold, or the Self, in Jungian terms. Therefore, it needs not to be slain. In a famous Chinese story of the Monkey King, Sun Wu-Kong, the white horse that was used to reach the final destiny, was actually a dragon. It was transmuted by the Buddha into a white horse for the sole purpose of accompanying the master on his journey. So, is it be possible that the inner dragon of me was transmuted into a horse (my Chinese affinity) in order for me to accomplish the tasks of this life's journey?

Some final thoughts

As my journey of studying the symbol of the dragon came to an end, I recalled a story that my 11-year-old therapy subject Zana told about a sand picture which she had constructed (Figure 7.12). In the sand picture, she placed a dragon, which she first called a demon, in the sand tray with a hand by the dragon's feet. She put a girl with her feet buried facing the dragon and a basket of eggs near the girl. Then, she placed a large lady at the lower right end of the tray who stood over the scene and watched. Zana told the following story about the tray:

> This girl was having a bad dream. A demon was coming behind her and a nest of eggs was by her. She was looking at the eggs, and while seeing the demon, her hand got caught in the nest. And then there was a voice. A lady telling her that she can control her own dreams, and that her arms will be free and that she can go to the demon. He will help her find her way home.

She further noted that the demon would kill and eat the people who don't control their dreams or are afraid of the demon. Based on her story, I was convinced that Zana, who had been sexually abused a few years prior to the therapy, was ready to take on the dragon, which represented the unconscious demon as well as the benevolent helper, and to be transformed.

As I pointed out earlier, in my own sandplay process, a horse appeared in an earlier tray whereas a dragon appeared in the last tray. Yes, my psychological need of integrating and transforming the horse and dragon seemed to have taken place in this sandplay process. Moreover, in this process of studying the dragon, I have felt like an alchemical dragon who was known to exist, destroy, and create; I have been transformed.

In conclusion, I would like to share an original poem about the dragon, written by Minna Hong, my dearest daughter and a great companion of this sandplay-book-journey:

> The dragon guards all he purviews
> He is fierce in his awesome majesty,
> A chimerical, whimsical creature
> He changes to fit each person's needs;
> In him, transformation is not
> Merely a possibility—it's inevitable.

Lastly, here is my dragon poem; it is the first poem that I have created in my life.

> Dragon, dragon, hero of my childhood fantasy
> Bright, shiny, beautiful, in ecstasy
> Dare or dare not, I chased you in my journey
> So glad that I found you in my reality!

Part IV

The author's sandplay research done in Taiwan

Part IV comprises the entire speech that I presented in the summer of 2005, at the International Society of Sandplay Therapy Congress at Zurich, Switzerland.

Chapter 11

Introduction

I am here with tremendous gratitude and humility to present my sandplay teaching experiences in Taiwan to you. I am grateful to all of you who have been there for me—my sandplay teachers, colleagues, the ISST, the STA, and my students. I am most thankful to the Garden of Hope Foundation in Taiwan of which I am a board member and an in-house professional consultant. The Garden of Hope Foundation provides me with the opportunity to teach sandplay and with the space—three sandplay teaching locations—for me to conduct workshops, seminars, and to administer sandplay processes. I am most humbled because I am truly more a novice than an experienced teacher, and I still have a lot to learn about sandplay.

I first learned about sandplay in 1991 when Barbara Weller, an ISST and STA Teaching Member, came to my graduate school, the Minnesota School of Professional Psychology, to give a brief introduction to sandplay. Ms. Weller was invited by my play therapy teacher, Dr. Jacquelyn Wiersma, and I instantly became attracted to this therapeutic mode. I felt it was my calling as a Christian, or my karma as the Asians say, or my *maktub* as the Arabians call it, to learn sandplay and to bring it to my native country, Taiwan. At that time, I was living in Minnesota. I embraced sandplay therapy fully, did my doctor degree (Psy.D.) dissertation on sandplay outcome research, and received my certificate from ISST and STA in 1996. For the next three years, I traveled to Taiwan, teaching sandplay on a short-term basis.

In December of 1999, I moved back to my native country, Taiwan, to teach sandplay on a more full-time basis. As time went on, more professional people in Taiwan were attracted to this therapeutic mode, and more and more students came to me for sandplay processes as well as for seminars and/or workshops. Currently, I have provided sandplay processes for around 150 people, and about 50 of them have completed their processes.

Challenges

As a solo teaching member in Taiwan, there are numerous challenges or difficulties. After I gave several introductory workshops, many professionals who attended were interested in taking personal processes. There isn't anyone else but me to provide this service. As time goes on, the waiting lists (at the three locations) have expanded and the wait time is longer (sometime it can be one to two years). So, my work time is expanding, and my health suffers because of it. Balancing the demands of learning the sandplay process that the numerous professionals have and providing the teaching of it in the limited amount of time I have is not an easy task. Through trial and error, I have learned the life lessons of limitations and, of course, patience.

When Dr. Hayao Kawai was invited to Taiwan to give talks and workshops last year, he told us that he had waited twenty years before he approved the formation of the sandplay association in Japan. Here in Taiwan, I did not wait twenty years, nor even five years, and agreed to form an association about three years ago [2002]. It was my intention to form an association that would make it easier to apply for grants and solicit help from the teachers in other countries. In that vein, we were able to get teachers from the United States and from Japan to come to Taiwan to teach sandplay. Thanks to all those who came. They gave valuable workshops, speeches, and consultations to sandplay students.

Despite the help, my workload drastically increased due to all the work related to forming the association. At my age, my body did not like the overwork and gave me a big warning sign. I got a serious stomach ulcer for the first time in my life shortly after the convention that we held last year. As a solo teacher, how I choose to spend my time becomes a great challenge. A related problem is the language barrier. Due to the cultural and language limitations, Taiwanese students are not very likely to go to teachers from another country to do their personal processes. So, I, knowing the languages and the culture here, am chosen to take this responsibility.

Still another challenge is the fact that no matter how many teachers we can afford to hire from abroad, I am the one who is here and expected to provide the processes, as well as workshops, seminars, and supervisions on a regular basis. It is difficult because in addition to the dual role of giving the processes and teaching, I have a third role that is either social or supervision-related to sandplay. Moreover, some students taking the processes are connected to each other, i.e., co-workers, classmates, or supervisors and employees. During the processes, they will talk about issues concerning their relationships. Keeping a proper objectivity about these issues is another challenge for me to face. In fact, some students taking processes from me are working under me. Even though I try to take every possible precaution to avoid boundary problems, I feel very uncomfortable with this issue at times. It is truly a great challenge to balance all these factors.

Rewards

As life continues, it seems that the more I face my challenges, the more rewards I reap. Perhaps one of the biggest rewards for me is the realization that there is life after age 60, a life that is full, challenging, and very meaningful. I have been truly blessed! No matter how difficult this life task is, I can always find the reward as well. With every sandplayer, the deeper the level of the psyche one delves into, the bigger is the treasure to be uncovered. All discoveries are not alike; they may be similar, but each is unique in its own way.

I rejoice as I witness the sandplayer's many accomplishments along the line. There is also tremendous joy when we, the sandplayer and I, jointly decide that the process is complete, and we celebrate it together. I cherish this moment as well as all the moments we have had together, knowing that we have, in this difficult life journey, shared many tears together, killed a few monsters, and harvested the fruits of life.

In order to share the joy of completing a sandplay process, I will show the final scenes of some of these brave life warriors. In addition, I have conducted a survey with them. Their views of the process will be shared as well.

Chapter 12

The sandplay outcome study of twelve professional mental health workers

Sandplayers

Our sandplayers consisted of twelve professional women who work in the mental health field and who have completed their sandplay processes recently, meaning in the past year or two. At the completion of the processes, their ages ranged from early thirties to late forties. The number of sandplay sessions they completed was twenty-four to eighty-two, whereas the number of sand pictures ranged from eleven to forty-six.

Final scenes

One or several of these themes were present in their final scenes:

1. Wholeness, centering, and unity
2. Returning to simplicity or nature, or back to real life
3. Serenity, peacefulness, and tranquility
4. Energy, movement, liveliness, and vitality
5. Completion, graduation, exiting, or journeying onward
6. Religion or spirituality
7. Softness, brightness, beauty, and colorfulness
8. Fruitfulness or abundance
9. Life-giving, growth or rebirth, and regeneration
10. Death and immortality
11. Family and togetherness
12. Joyfulness, festivity, and celebration

Next, I would like to present the sandplayers' final scenes. For identification purposes, I will call them Subject 1 through Subject 12.

Subject 1's final sand picture

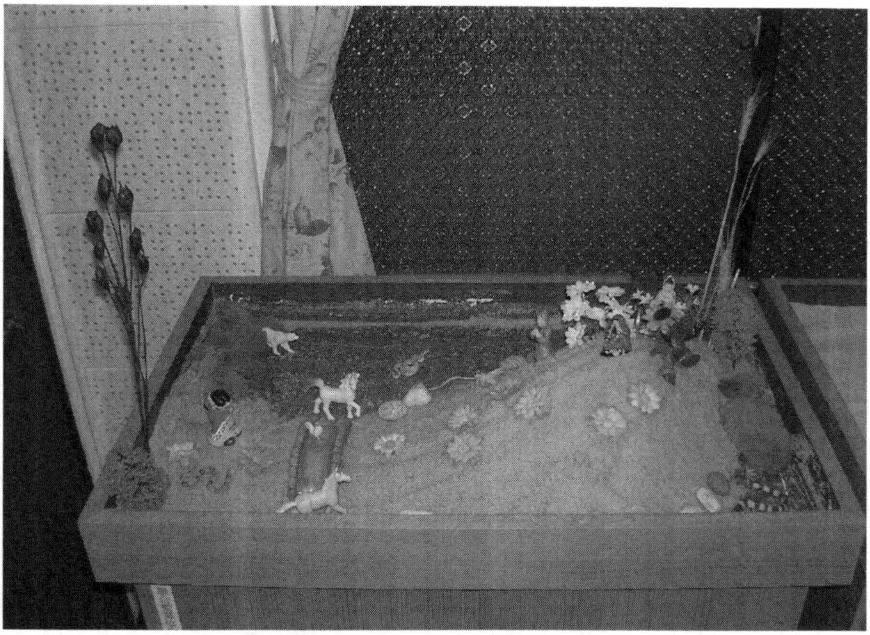

Figure 12.1 Subject 1's final sand picture.

Subject 1 made a rather beautiful and lively final scene (Figure 12.1). In the upper right corner, Guan Yin and the storyteller, situated on top of the hill in the midst of flowers with a monk standing nearby, seemed to be protecting and blessing the whole universe. Flowers were plentiful, as were trees and crops. Snakes, roaming here and there over the tray, including the one near the native girl that was identified by Subject 1 as herself, seemed to signify both destructive and regenerative powers. Subject 1 noted that this girl was not afraid of the snake. A chicken, also designated as representing Subject 1 (she was born in the Year of the Chicken), crossing a bridge near the lower left corner, was protected by two galloping unicorns. Another bridge, located on the ridge of the tray near the upper right corner, seemed to represent the journey onward into the mystery future.

Overall, themes of beauty, liveliness, abundance, regeneration, and journeying onward are apparent.

Subject 2's final sand picture

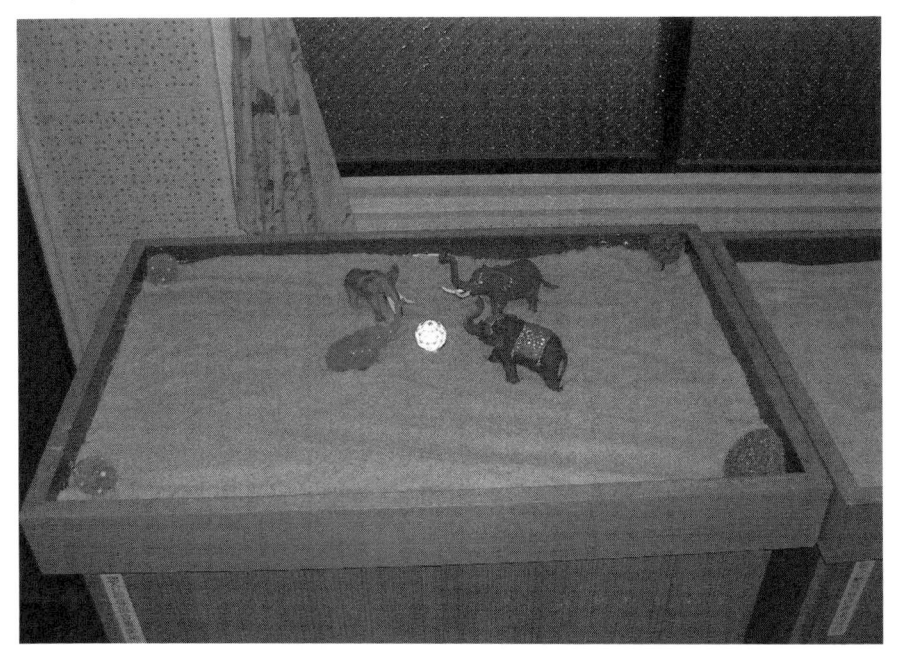

Figure 12.2 Subject 2's final sand picture.

In this final scene (Figure 12.2), Subject 2 kept it very simple: four trees, one in each outer corner and four elephants near the center, surrounding a centered crystal ball. She noted that the four elephants were lifting the centered ball as if lifting the whole universe, carrying hope with them.

Themes of wholeness and completion represented by the repetition of the number four; centering, simplicity, and energy and vitality are present.

Sandplay study of twelve mental health workers 123

Subject 3's final sand picture

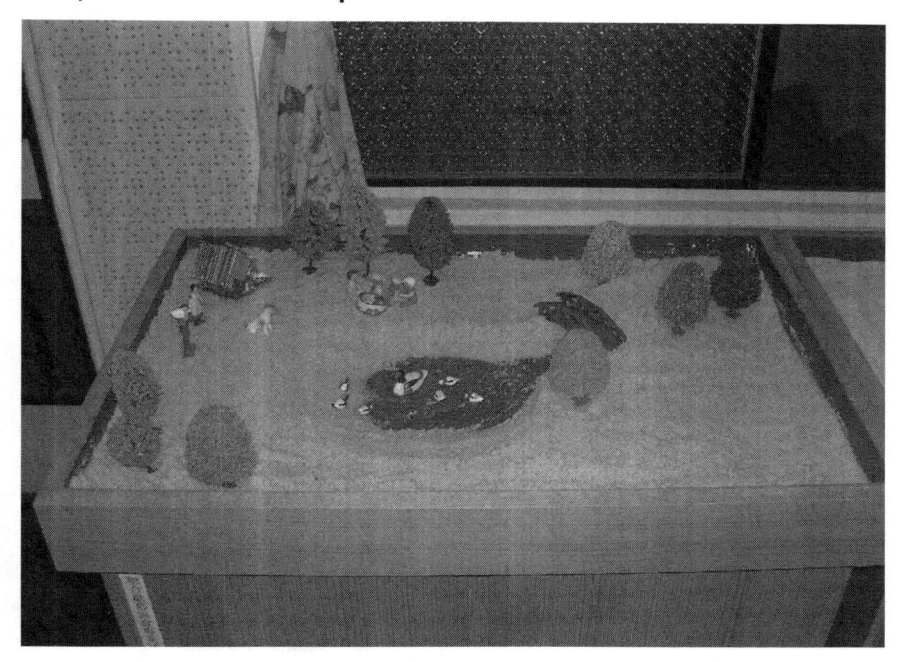

Figure 12.3 Subject 3's final sand picture.

Subject 3 created a very peaceful family scene (Figure 12.3) in her final session. In this picture, the members of a duck family swam in or played near the lake in the center, whereas a family of people plus their dog were placed outside of their family home. Children happily played, and food was nearby. The children's working parents appeared watchful and protective a short distance away. Colorful trees and a bridge were placed around the people and ducks, giving the impression of serenity and fruitfulness.

In addition to themes of peacefulness and serenity, centering, family and togetherness, colorfulness and fruitfulness, the themes of returning to simplicity and nature and back to real life are evident.

Subject 4's final sand pictures

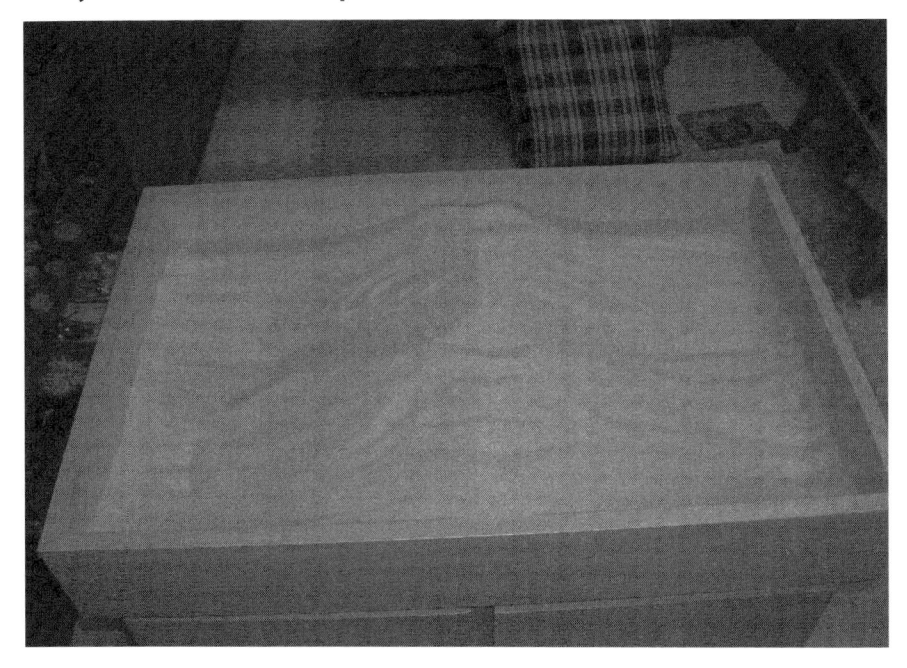

Figure 12.4a Subject 4's final sand picture (dry tray).

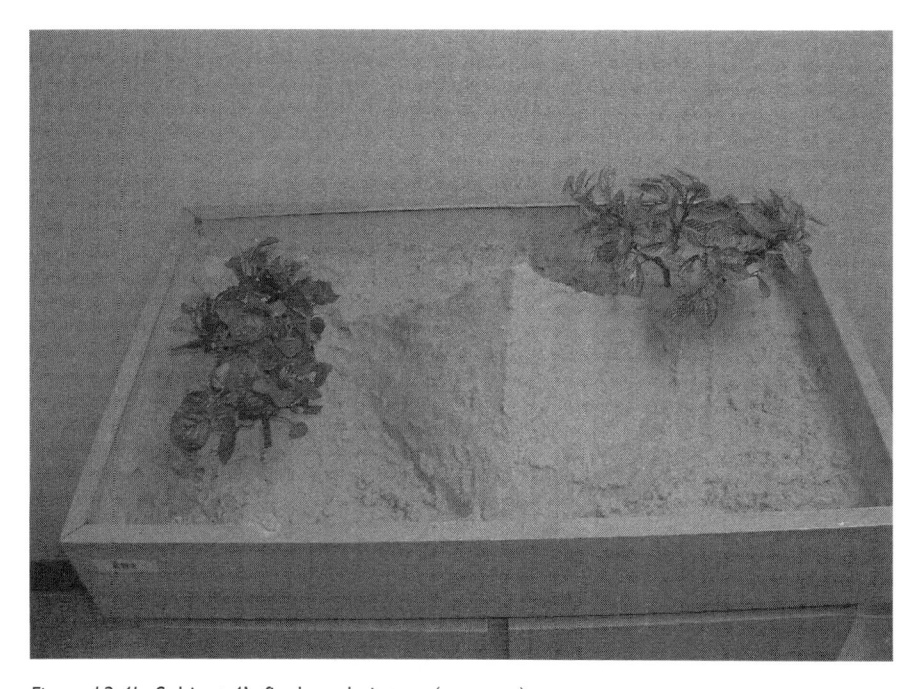

Figure 12.4b Subject 4's final sand picture (wet tray).

In her final session, Subject 4 made two sand scenes. Both were simple and beautiful. In the dry tray (Figure 12.4a), she used all the sand and made a large and distinctive face. It was very artistic. Upon finishing, she commented that it could be either the sun god or the wind god. The face was known to be a deity image and God's protection, as noted by Ad de Vries (1984, p. 174). In the wet tray (Figure 12.4b), Subject 4 pushed most of the sand into the center and molded it into a three-sided pyramid before placing large trees in the upper right and lower left corners. She seemed rather pleased with the outcome and commented: "I was making a pyramid. While I was making it, I thought the sand was really a wonderful and meaningful thing."

A pyramid is known to signify death and immortality, whereas a tree often represents growth, perpetual regeneration, victory over death, and immortality. Thus, themes of returning to simplicity, spirituality, death and immortality, and growth and regeneration are present in these two final scenes.

Subject 5's final sand picture

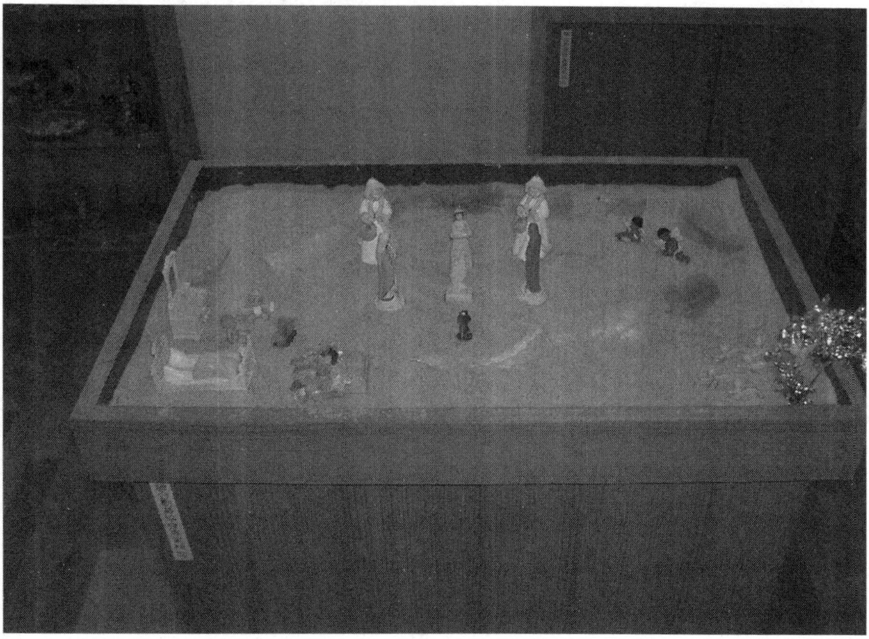

Figure 12.5 Subject 5's final sand picture.

In Subject 5's rather serene, soft, and centered scene (Figure 12.5), the blessing and celebration of the new-born baby held by the mother near the center was represented by the centered praying hands. The praying hands were surrounded by a circle of two St. Mary figures, the twin-women, the silver family sculpture, and the little female silver figure blowing a flute.

Furthermore, the presence of twin angels in the upper right corner and many little angels located under and in the silver tree near the lower right corner reinforced the theme of joyfulness and blessings. In the lower left corner, two babies, surrounded by furniture, a toy train, and an opened gift box, were playing. A circle of feathers was located in the outer skirt, giving an impression of softness and colorfulness.

Overall, this final scene reflects themes of centering, spirituality, life-giving, peacefulness and serenity, joyfulness and celebration, and softness and colorfulness.

Subject 6's final sand picture

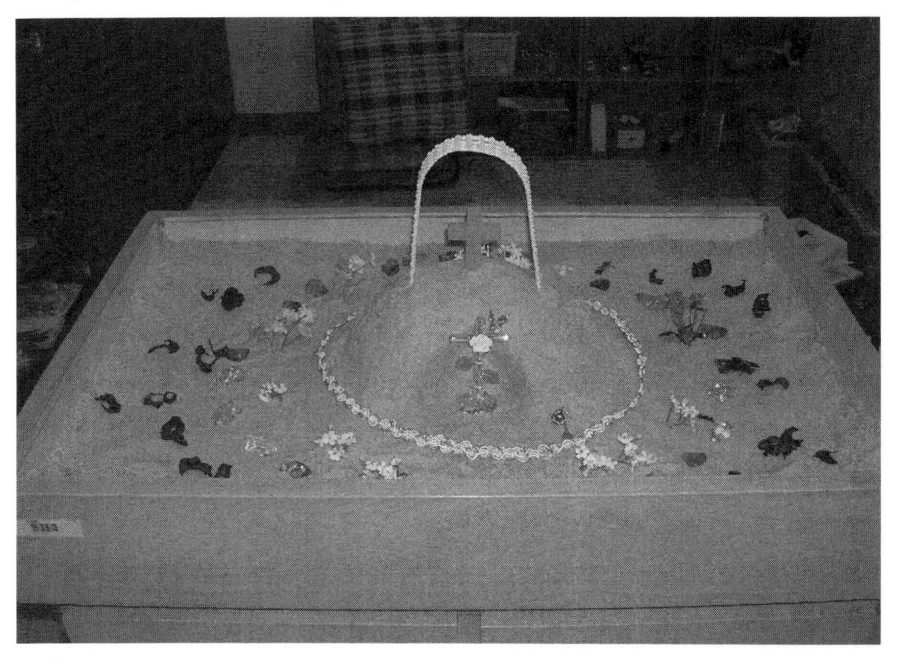

Figure 12.6 Subject 6's final sand picture.

In Subject 6's rather simple scene (Figure 12.6), a cross with a dove on the top right of it and a rose plant growing in the center of the cross was placed right at the entrance of a small cave. The cave was located at the bottom of a hill. Subject 6 made the hill in the center of the tray. The bottom of the hill was bordered with a circle of interlaced flowers. A white gate was placed on top of the hill, and another cross stood right under the gate. On the outskirts of the whole center scene, pieces of dried flowers and colorful flat marbles were scattered. About this final scene, Subject 6 commented that what was buried was now open and that there was a flower (rose) on the cross, signifying a life that was colorful, creative, and growing, and a life that was capable of creating more lives.

According to J.C. Cooper (1979, p. 141), the rose is both heavenly perfection and earthly passion. In addition, he noted that in the symbolism of the heart, the rose occupies the central point of the cross, the point of unity. In this tray, outside of the rose that is located in the center, another rose is placed in a golden vase and located in the lower right of the cross, reinforcing the same theme. Overall, themes of centering, unity, tranquility, spirituality, rebirth and regeneration, and simplicity and colorfulness are present.

Subject 7's final sand picture

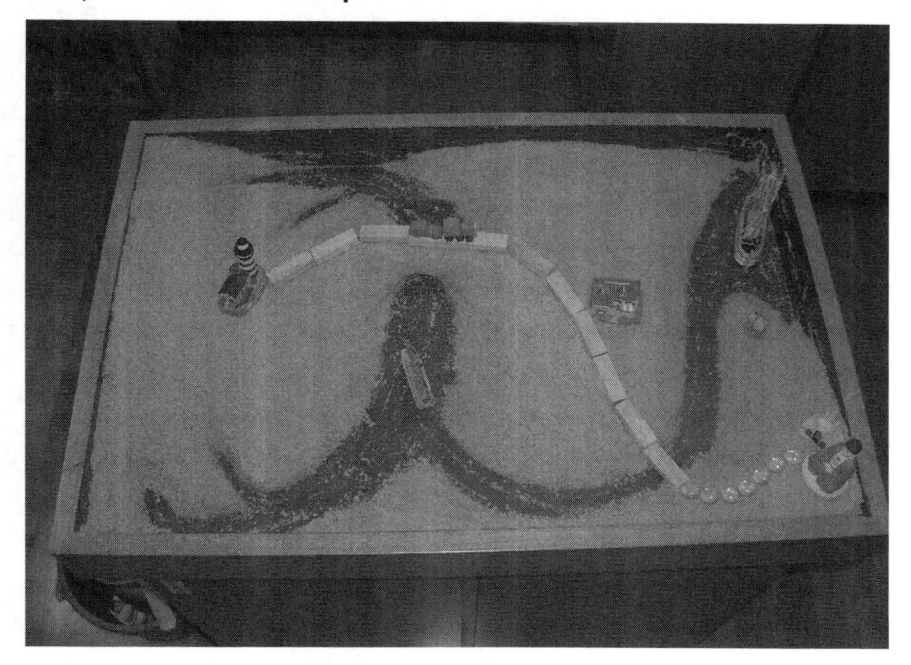

Figure 12.7 Subject 7's final sand picture.

In Subject 7's final scene (Figure 12.7), perhaps the most salient feature was the representation of movement. A train was moving in the direction of the church and the Buddha, and two boats were sailing with one crossing through a tunnel. Moreover, the blue at the bottom of the tray that was supposed to be the stream or the water was shaped like a huge flying bird, ready to take it all and fly away.

Themes of journeying onward, vitality and movement, and spirituality and brightness are present. Brightness is represented by the lighthouse.

Subject 8's final sand picture

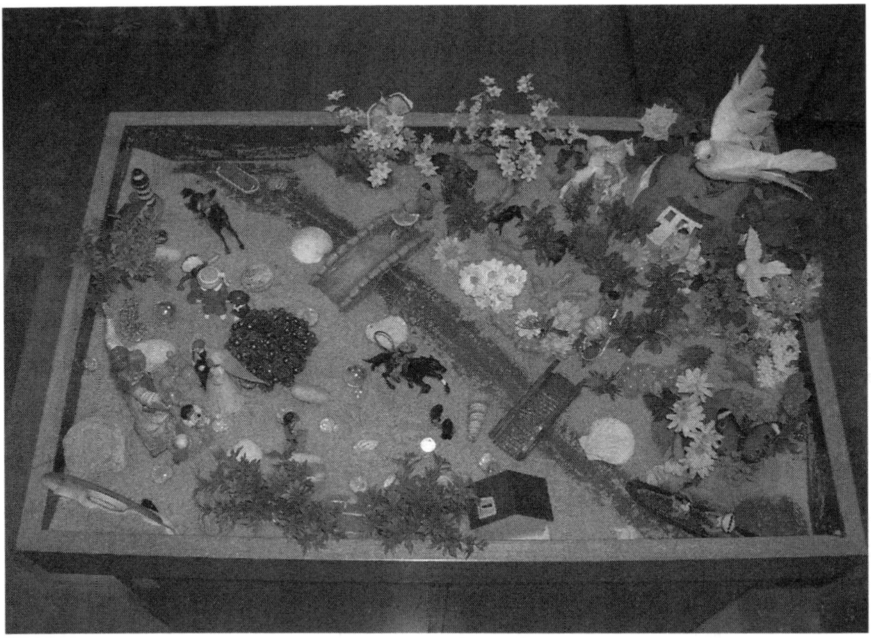

Figure 12.8 Subject 8's final sand picture.

Subject 8 produced a beautiful, colorful scene (Figure 12.8) that was full of life. There were lots of flowers, trees, and bushes as well as rocks, flat colorful glass marbles, pine cones, and dried flowers. A stream ran from the top left corner of the tray to the lower right with two bridges connecting the two sides and a lighthouse at the top end. A huge white bird stood on a beautiful sky dome, and a small white bird and a big flying owl were nearby.

Standing in front of the dome was Guan Yin, a Chinese goddess who was known to bless childbirth and to protect all children. Opposite her, in the far left lower corner, was a huge statue of Jesus, raising his arms in a gesture of blessing. A rainbow sat right behind him. A newlywed couple and several children, a mother and a child, and an Indian male, seemingly blissful, were placed in front of Jesus. A canoe, guided by an Indian chief, was moving from the bottom right toward the top left. Another boat, situated at the top left, was ready to sail. Two horseback riders galloped through the lower field, whereas a man and a woman, each pushing a wheelbarrow loaded with watermelons, were about to cross the bridges. There were plenty of animals, freely roaming. Fruits were plentiful as well.

In this final scene, themes of spirituality and unity are symbolized by the presence of both Guan Yin and Jesus. In addition, the highly elevated flying white bird seems to signify the presence of the Holy Spirit that is watchful, protective, and active. The theme of liveliness or vitality is shown by the galloping horseback riders and the hard-working man and woman who are preparing to cross the bridges, as well as by the free-roaming animals. The spirituality theme is again present in the blessing of Jesus of the newlywed couple, children, and everyone else. The theme of journeying onward is reflected vividly in many parts of this picture and in particular by the canoeists and the horseback riders. Moreover, themes of serenity, fruitfulness and abundance, and colorfulness and brightness are shown in all parts of this picture. All in all, this is truly a blissful scene that is full of the aforementioned themes.

Subject 9's final sand picture

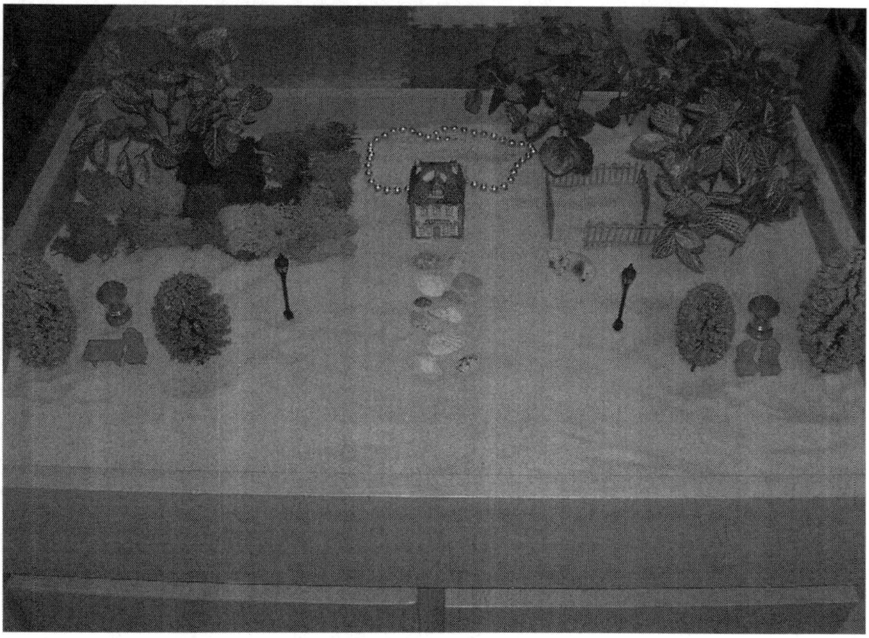

Figure 12.9 Subject 9's final sand picture.

Subject 9 built a "home" for her final scene (Figure 12.9). According to her, this was "my home." In her home, there were dogs, and the living quarter for the dogs was nearby. She also placed trees so that their shade protected her home. In the backyard, there was a dirt ground for children to play in, and in front, there was a walking trail and benches for pedestrians to rest on as needed. Street lights were present, too.

Overall, themes of returning to simplicity and nature, back to real life, brightness, family and togetherness, and peacefulness are evident in this final scene.

Subject 10's final sand picture

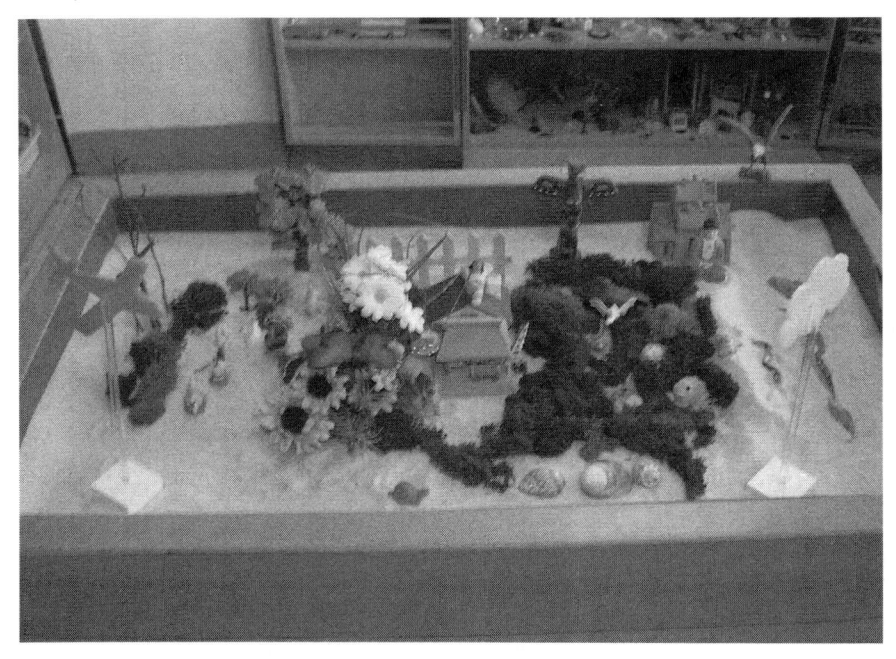

Figure 12.10 Subject 10's final sand picture.

In Subject 10's final scene (Figure 12.10), a peaceful and relaxed country life was depicted. A girl, lying down and situated on top of the roof, seemed rather relaxed. Two houses next to each other and located in the center of the tray were surrounded with lots of greenery, shells, and colorful flowers. Dogs, frogs, a snake, a snail, a school of fish, domestic birds, and wild birds were scattered throughout this natural environment. Clouds, an airplane, and an eagle were in the air, signifying free-flowing energy. A totem pole and a temple with a Buddha sitting in front of the temple, located in the outskirts, seemed to be providing protection for all.

In all, the themes of returning to simplicity and nature, back to real life, serenity and peacefulness, and spirituality are indicated.

Subject 11's final sand picture

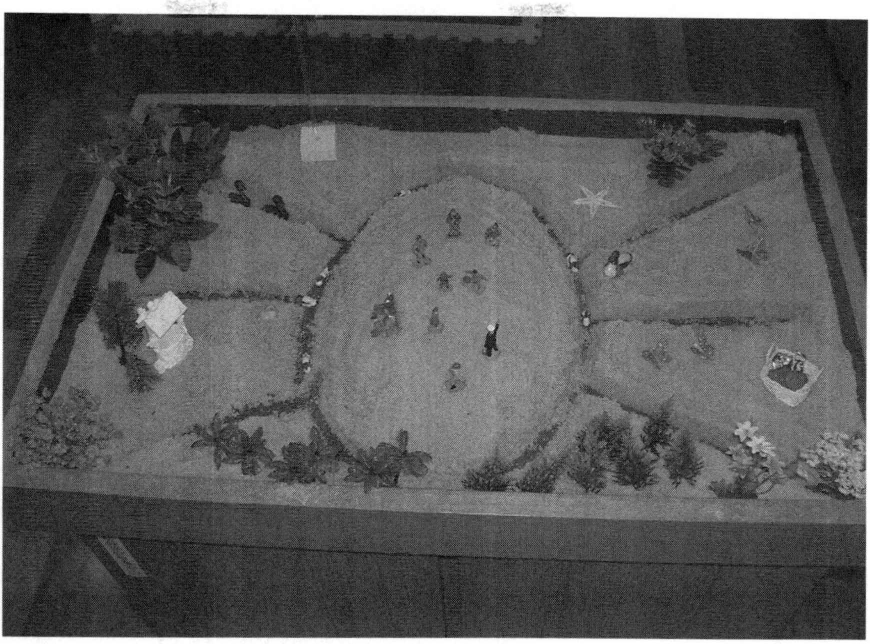

Figure 12.11 Subject 11's final sand picture.

Subject 11's final scene (Figure 12.11) looked simple, and yet centered, colorful, bright and lively. Brightness was shown in the radiating shape of the whole center, which was at ground level and reinforced itself with the sunlight, radiating from the top left corner (not seen in this picture). In the centred island, people were relaxed, at ease, and friendly. Peacefulness was displayed by the ducks swimming around the circular stream, guarded by the mother duck in the upper right corner just outside of the centred island. Peacefulness was also represented by the swans that were freely floating in the stream and by the butterflies that were also peacefully resting on the right side of the tray. Both people and animals were free, and yet seemed together—imparting a sense of serenity. The trees and flowers were blooming. The life energy was supplied by the light and the water coming both from the well that was situated in the lower left corner and by the streams.

Two key-and-lock figures were resting in the basket in the lower right corner. The sandplayer commented that they represented the therapist and the sandplayer. Together, she said, they unlocked something, perhaps the mystery of life. The centred island was in the shape of an egg, and the whole picture was in the shape of a scarab; they appear to signify rebirth and regeneration.

Overall, this final scene reflects themes of wholeness, centering and unity, brightness and colorfulness, peacefulness and serenity, and rebirth and regeneration.

Subject 12's final sand picture

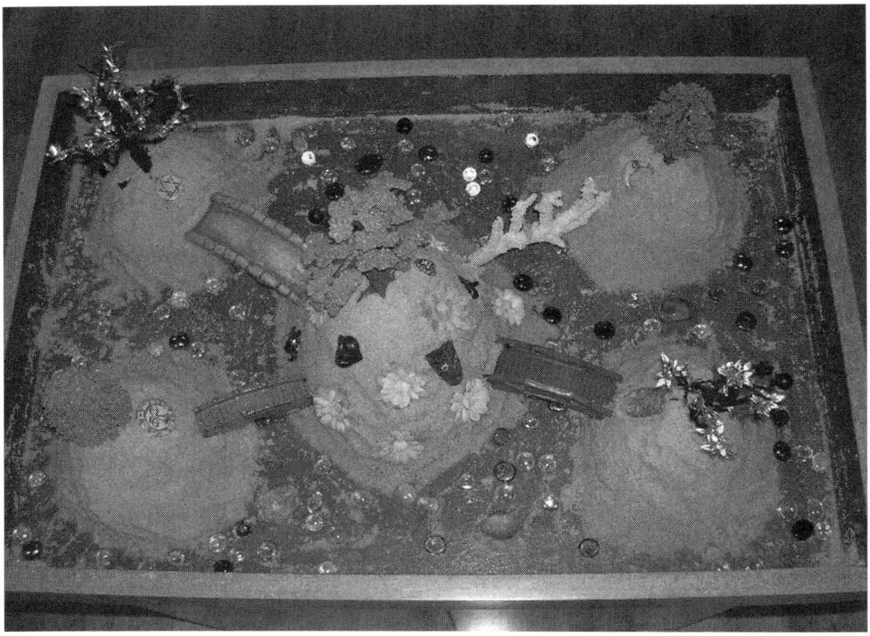

Figure 12.12 Subject 12's final sand picture.

In this final scene of Subject 12 (Figure 12.12), the most salient features were the presence of the number four and the number five. There were four bridges, four ivory disks (in the shapes of a sun, a moon, a star, and a face) located on the surface of four outer mounds (one disk on each mound), five total mounds, five trees, and five masks located on the centered mound.

The number four is known to symbolize wholeness, totality, and completion, whereas the number five is often associated with the center of the integration of – or the center that is connecting – the four directions, representing universality. Therefore, themes of wholeness, unity, and completion are indicated.

Another notable theme is rebirth and regeneration. This is reflected in the growth of silver and golden branches on the seemingly dead, barren, black trees located in the upper left and lower right corners and by the many colorful flowers on the surface of the center mound. The many shiny flat glass marbles scattered on the surface of the blue ocean seemed to be radiating light. An oak tree stood upright in the center of the whole tray, signifying strength and vitality.

Overall, themes of wholeness, unity, completion, brightness, colorfulness, rebirth and regeneration, and vitality are present.

Survey results

There are two parts to this survey, as shown in the Appendix. Please see the Appendix for the categories used, which are capitalized below. Here are the results for the first part:

1 Approximately three-quarters of the participants stated that their sandplay processes have had a positive impact on their Emotional Stability, Self-Confidence, Objective Awareness of Events in Life, Psychological Energy, and Spiritual Growth.
2 Approximately one-half of the participants checked that their sandplay processes have had a positive impact on their Self-Concept/Image, Inter-Personal Relationships, Problem-Solving Ability, and Independence and Self-Assertion.
3 Approximately one-third indicated that their sandplay processes have had a significant and positive impact in the areas of Communication and Expressive Ability, Cognitive and Logic Ability, Frustration Tolerance, and Sense of Responsibility.
4 Approximately one-quarter reported that the sandplay process has had a positive impact in the area of Physical Health.
5 Other areas that have been positively impacted, noted by single individuals, are: Relationship with Family Members and Attachment, Integration of Femininity and Masculinity, and Trauma Recovery.

In the second part, this question was raised: "Within one hundred words, please state your thoughts and feelings about completing the sandplay process." Here are their statements:

Subject 1

When doing a sand tray, my inner thoughts or unconscious are likely to be projected onto the miniatures that I placed in the tray. Not consciously knowing what I was doing, I became clearer about my inner world and in touch with my inner strength. With the presence of the therapist, I was able to complete the process in a free and protected atmosphere.

Subject 2

I do not know how the process will evolve in the future. However, I am most impressed with my first and last sand pictures. The last sand picture has been my source of encouragement.

Subject 3

During the process, many times I was truly resistant. I did not know whether I was resistant to facing myself or the therapist. However, when I overcame my resistance, some incredible sand pictures occurred, and they often reflected my inner world. Moreover, several times during the process, the synchronicity events as described by Jung appeared, and I was amazed. Overall, the biggest impact or my most important accomplishments that I have gotten from the process are the elevation of my self-concept and the resolution of a life trauma that occurred early in my life.

Subject 4

I feel that this is a very important life experience. I went from doubting the existence of an unconscious world to becoming amazed by it, realizing that it is life's elementary energy. Not needing words, the unconscious energy was invoked; it was purer and more direct. It was truly an indescribable wonder! Now, devoting myself to giving sandplay therapy has become my career goal.

Subject 5

In the protective environment of sandplay, it was quite safe to communicate with my inner self. Thus, I have re-found my psychological inner power, and have more capacity to face and solve life problems.

Subject 6

Through the work of sandplay and dream analysis, I have experienced much inner transformation. In theory, it may be called self-integration. Moreover, I am more accepting of my shadow, and I like myself much better. In better understanding myself, I have changed, not only in the way I treat myself, but also in the way I am with my spouse and my family of origin.

Subject 7

The sand pictures will reappear in my daily life and bring me energy. With the progression of the sandplay therapy, I feel myself becoming more stable, and I can see the growth. I do not understand how it occurs, but I truly feel that I have become more of an independent, self-assertive, and self-responsible individual.

Subject 8

Upon completing the process, I feel my biggest accomplishment is the re-establishment of contact with myself. Everything feels real now, I am in touch; I can see; I can feel. It is so nice to be able to feel life. A miracle has happened to me. It is like a curse being lifted off a princess; I am alive!

Subject 9

The sandplay process has been a miraculous experience. It has helped me release my emotions and has brought me the kind of happiness that comes from the bottom of my heart. I have seen my creativity and felt proud of my accomplishments.

Subject 10

At first, I was motivated to do sandplay because of my curiosity. I did not have any clue about my unconscious. I did not consider myself as a person with problems and did not accept my real senses and feelings. Even though I had been in the mental health field for many years, I was fearful of getting in touch with my inner wounds. As I progressed through my process, I found that every part of me was yelling at myself to reflect. I began to realize that there was an inner self and inner energy. I experienced more and more awareness and transformation. Every time I realized a different awareness, my vision of inner self expanded incredibly.

Subject 11

As an adult, I was seeking a secure and free space. Through the therapist's warm and consistent protecting and accompaniment, I have had a chance to sink and re-grow. It is truly a unique experience. Every time I see what I previously did not see in myself, it is truly moving and precious. The source or the energy of life has now been expanding.

Subject 12

Subject 12 did a rather lengthy report. In essence, she stated that at the time when she entered the process, she was in turmoil. Making a sand tray often brought her great joy. "Every time I finished a tray, I loved to stand in front of it, appreciating what I had made. Seeing the inner self concretely appear, I often felt greatly moved." She noted that she began to accept herself, to discover new things and even to try new things. She has changed. She even overcame her fear of snakes. At the time of completion, she felt confident about herself, emotionally more stable, and had a better relationship with her father, who she felt had traumatized her in her early life. She concluded:

> I am most thankful to my therapist who was always genuine. During the sandplay process, she provided me a free and protective space. I felt safe to say and do anything. I have gotten a lot and feel that it (the process) will be the important life spring of my future.

Conclusion

In all, my experience of being a solo sandplay teaching member in Taiwan has been full of great challenges and incredible rewards. I have become more aware of my limitations and the limitations of life itself in general, and yet, at the same time, I am more confident of the unlimited potential that I have and that life can provide. Of course, the sandplay practice and teaching have been a great part of this discovery. At this point, I would like to say that I owe much of it to my students—the sandplayers in this study. They have had the patience and the courage to endure the challenges of their sandplay processes with me. They are truly my teachers! Lastly, I thank the almighty God who has given me a chance to do this work and who has protected me all the way. Praise the Lord!

Part V

The author's sandplay case done in Taiwan

Chapter 13

Introduction of the case

Jade, a middle-aged married woman, mother of two children, and a professional, casually walked into the sandplay therapy room several years ago. She smiled shyly and told me that the reasons she came were similar to those of other professionals; she wanted to advance in her counseling professional career, to learn sandplay, and to understand herself. When she was asked specifically if she had any personal problems, she replied that she sometimes had low moods and occasional temper flare-ups. With such a brief and seemingly non-alarming introduction, she and I became engaged in a long-term sandplay process that was filled with dangers, anxieties, and challenges. Nevertheless, it also became unusually fruitful, productive, and transforming.

During the initial stage, there appeared to be the presence of creative regression in that she, upon touching the sand and miniatures, became quite regressive and became aware of her earlier traumatic life experiences. In fact, she was very suicidal for a certain period, and I had to use active strategies, i.e., non-suicide contract, and other resources, in order to protect her from committing suicide and me from anxiety.

Throughout the sandplay process, especially during the initial stage, Jade would become very upset about the fact that she could not find her feelings, thus, she would not know how to do a sand tray. At those moments, sometimes she would say, "I might as well kill myself." Significantly, toward the end of the process, she commented, "I am so happy that I found myself," or, "I am home!" Jade, a brave life warrior, at the end of the process said that she felt proud that she challenged her life and that she had risen above, felt stable, very reaffirmed, and saw the covenant. She added that it was truly a worthwhile process.

In approximately four years, Jade did eighty-two sessions. Normally, I provided only twenty sessions per year for my sandplay professional students because of the limitations of my time. However, when Jade suffered from acute severe depression, I extended my limits and gave her extra sessions. Jade did a total of forty-five sand pictures. While her sand trays were infrequent during the initial stage, toward the end of the process, she did one tray almost every session. In fact, she became very attached to the sand trays and experienced anxiety over terminating therapy. Steps were taken in order to prepare her for termination.

In Chapter 14, I will share her twenty-four sand trays, give each tray a title, and describe the sand tray making process. In addition, I have included Jade's comments about her pictures and my interpretations of these pictures. I will also briefly share the contents of omitted pictures in order to give a sense of continuity concerning the process. Because of the fact that Jade tends to use many miniatures in each tray, I cannot note or comment on every item, nor interpret each of them. So, I hope you will use your intuition, your knowledge about symbols, and your wisdom to make sense out of the ones I don't mention.

At this point, I'd like to invite the reader again, as I did in the chapter about Zana, to hold Jade in your heart, silently blessing her to have better psychological health, growth, and integrity. I deeply thank her for her willingness to consent to my going public with her case.

Chapter 14

Jade's sandplay rebirth process
From darkness to light

Sand picture 1

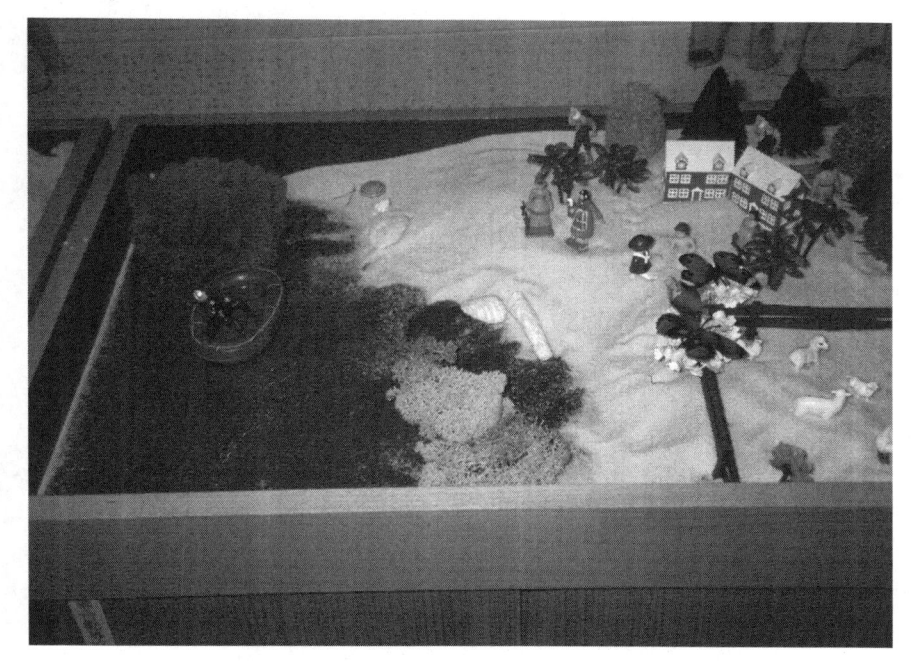

Figure 14.1 The me who is lost.

Sand tray making process

Jade used the dry sand for this tray (Figure 14.1). While she was pushing most of the sand from the right side to the left, she commented: "The sand is too much!" When told that she could take out some sand, she did. Then she placed two houses in the upper right corner and surrounded them with some trees. Immediately after, she built a fence around the lower right corner and placed domestic animals there, including two horses, two chickens, three lambs, and one goat (some are not shown in this picture). In front and in back of the house, she placed working men and women, two small children, and a dog. To the left, she placed a man with an oar in a life raft drifting in the sea, surrounded by chunks of sea reefs and shells around the shore. At the end of the session, she placed flowers around the fence and two huge butterflies on the flowers.

Jade's comments

Upon finishing the tray, Jade said: "Many items that I wanted are not here. Those people are not what I wanted, neither are the trees. The butterflies are too big, and so are the flowers. The only thing that makes me feel right is the diligent work by the workers."

Therapist's interpretations

In the beginning, Jade's negative comments on how she felt there were an insufficient number of miniatures at the therapist's office were significant; she readily showed her negative transference toward the therapist. Her criticism might have meant, "The mom is bad. She does not know my needs!" Jade's ability to show her dissatisfaction, however, is a good sign, suggesting her willingness to engage in the process in spite of her negative feelings.

Generally speaking, the client's first tray tells of his or her problems as well as speaks to the prognosis. In this tray, the drastic difference between what seems to be a pleasant country scene and a rather dark, stark, ominous seashore scene suggests the extreme opposite of her two selves that are perhaps split—an apparently normal self and an emotional self that seems lonely, alienated, and in danger. Similarly, the polarity of self is reflected on the right side; adults are working, whereas children are sitting by themselves, and the animals are completely fenced off with no food and no door. The darkness or the depression of the client is vividly shown by the man on the raft who is surrounded by sea reefs. He is all alone, seems stuck, and perhaps feels like drowning, and no help is in sight.

The diligent working of adults seems to reflect her avoidance defense, and perhaps is representing the part of self that is desperately trying to stay healthy. She perhaps numbs herself, dissociating from her feelings, diligently working to avoid her troublesome inner shadowy self.

On the positive side, Jade's willingness to dig out the sand and make a water scene is a good sign. That is an indication that she wants to be in touch with her unconscious, no matter how frightening it can be. The possibility to integrate the polarity of the dark and light, or in an Asian term, the yin and yang appears to be the task at hand.

Sand picture 2

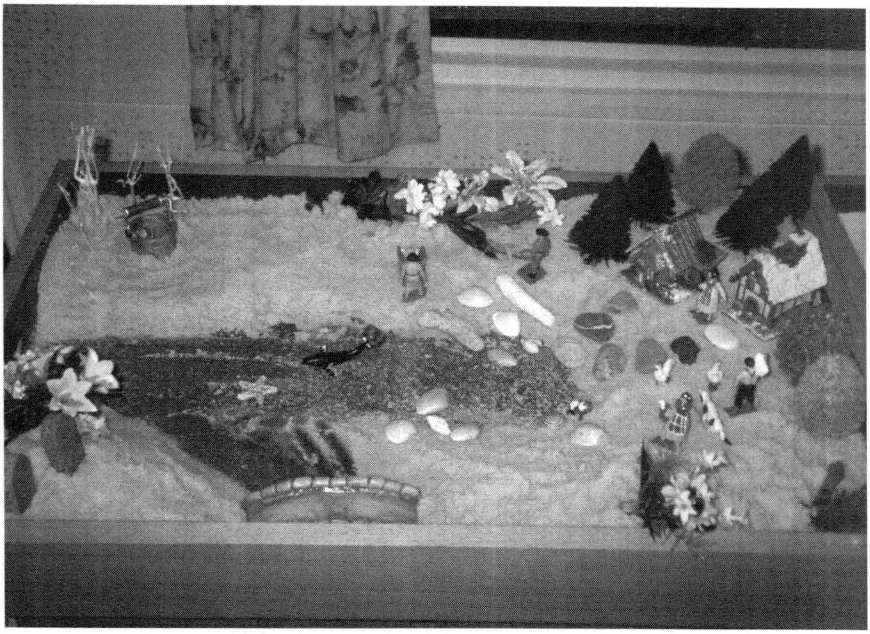

Figure 14.2 Who is or are under the tombstones?

Sand tray making process

Before she made the tray (Figure 14.2), Jade told me that she had had a dream the previous night. In this dream, she was bravely swimming (Jade was afraid of swimming). In contrast to the previous tray, Jade used wet sand for this tray. She first dug out some sand and made a water scene. She then placed a bridge between the lower left land and the land on the right. The bridge spanned the stream and connected the land of people to the land of the dead—the graveyard. She put a small whale, a small starfish, and shells in the water, and some more shells, stones, a little swan, and a glass frog along the shore. On the right side, there was a country scene: there were two houses, trees and flowers, working adults, two chickens, and a running dog. In the upper left corner, there was a well and its bucket; the well is placed near many dried branches. In the lower left corner, two erect tombstones were placed among some colorful flowers.

Jade's comments

Upon completion of the scene, Jade said:

> I really do not like to put this bridge, but it has to be there. The tombstones have to be there, and the flowers, too. Of course, the working people must be there. I do not know who is or who are under the tombstones. If it is me, then I hope there will be more flowers. The branches [upper left] are drying, and the water of the well may make them green again.

Therapist's interpretations

During the initial stage of the sandplay therapy process, the trays may indicate what the client's problems are and from where these problems come. In this tray, the upper left corner's very dried branches and the barrenness suggest the possibility of early deprivation, whereas the presence of the well with its bucket indicates the remedy. Furthermore, the graveyard in the lower left corner mirrors the desire in her to bury or forget her early childhood that was probably quite barren and unbearable. Interestingly, she placed two tombstones plus several pairs of items in the first and second trays—perhaps reflecting twin parts of herself or her need to have a companion.

The connecting bridge between the present (the right, her seemingly normal side) and the past (the left, representing the dark side of her) was placed in the tray reluctantly by the client. Nevertheless, it represents her ambivalent willingness to dig deep and integrate her shadow with her consciousness.

In the water and at the center of the tray, a swimming black whale seems to represent the psycho pomp, her energy and guiding force, bravely swimming toward the dark unconscious of her past. It mirrors her dream of getting into water and swimming. The starfish, of course, could be the link between the heaven and the sea—with the star illuminating the way for her. The little swan, the little frog, and two butterflies from the first tray are all transforming symbols, pointing out the possibility for her to transcend herself.

Sand picture 3

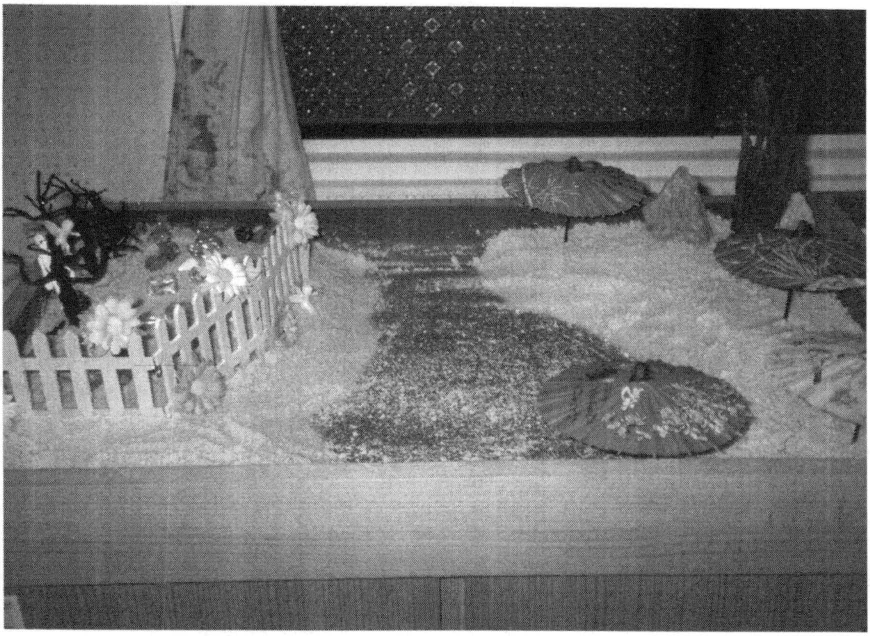

Figure 14.3 My tomb.

Prior to this session, Jade did not make a tray for several sessions and neither did she do so after a summer break of nearly two months. During the verbal part of our session, she told me that as a child she was scolded many times and told to go kill herself. She felt very unwanted. Suicidal thoughts were present both as a child and an adolescent. Recently, she again had suicidal thoughts. In the beginning of this session, she struggled a bit about making a tray, feeling quite uneasy and somewhat frightened. Upon further discussion, she made up her mind and said, "I am going to make a tomb for myself."

Sand tray making process

In the middle, there was a vase-shaped pond, separating two lands, one on the right and one on the left (Figure 14.3). There was a narrow connection between the two lands (not shown in this picture) at the bottom. Jade buried a huge casket (unseen in this picture) in the left land where two dead trees and two skeletons (a black one and a white one) were standing. Hanging on a dead tree was a small angel. Several other small angels were scattered either on the edge or on the fence that Jade built around the graveyard. Many colorful glass stones were scattered on the grave ground. Flowers were hung on the fence. In the right land, four large, colorful, opened umbrellas were placed. In the upper right corner, a huge piece of cedar wood was placed in an upright position, and a small mountain-shaped stone was set on each side of the piece of wood.

Jade's comments

Jade said:

> I feel much better now. I like both sides. I am glad that I let myself die [in the tray], but I do not want to have a tombstone. Letting myself die gave me good feelings . . . Dying in the sand tray is safer. However, I do not know how many more times that I will have to die [in the tray].

She added that she was very suicidal the previous day, but felt good that she did not do it because she enjoyed the presence of today.

Therapist's interpretations

The near lack of connection between the two sides is alarming. However, the narrow connecting line of sand at the bottom indicates a slight possibility and hope of integration. The little hanging angel, the presence of a huge buried casket, two dead trees, and two skeletons all point to a severe and active depression. On the other hand, the protective power of the right side, represented by the umbrellas and the upright piece of cedar wood, suggests some hopeful signs. However, would that be enough? Is there a chance that the client will be successful in committing suicide? At this critical stage of the process, I took active suicidal preventive strategies, including asking her to see a psychiatrist to determine a need for medication, making a non-suicide contract, and giving her extra sessions.

Sand picture 4

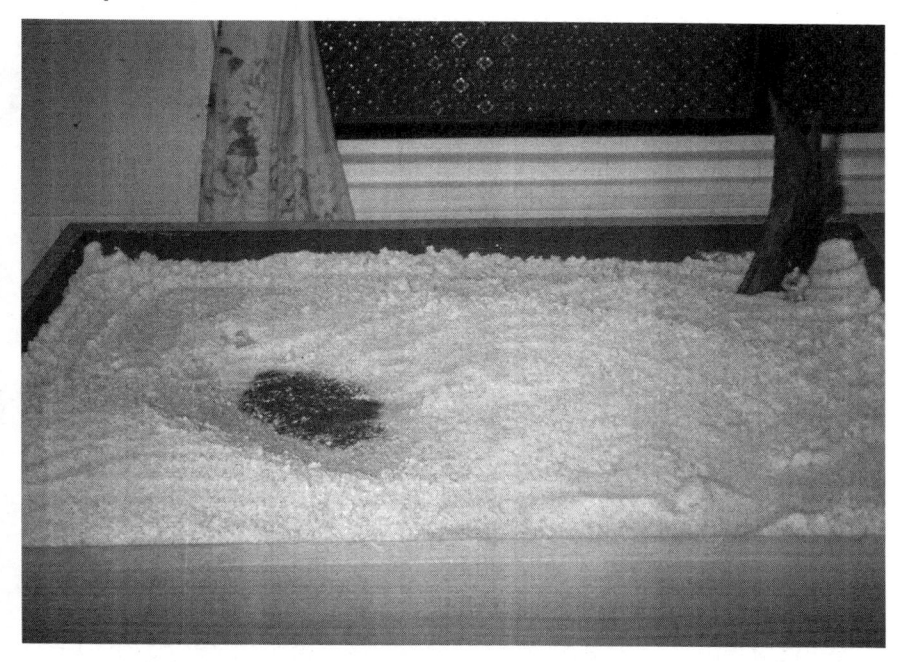

Figure 14.4 Vast depression and a breathing oasis.

Sand tray making process

Upon arrival, Jade immediately went to work on the sand (Figure 14.4). She made a small opening on the left side of the tray and erected the cedar wood in the upper right corner. She then selected a Native American mother holding a baby and placed it near the hole before initiating an attempt to bury the figure. She changed her mind and moved the figure, placed it under the cedar wood, instead.

Jade's comments

In tears Jade said, "This is my current feeling—very afraid to come here because I became aware of the fact that I am no good. I hate myself and want to bury myself, just be dead." She added that she had devoted herself to Buddhism, studying it, actively worshipping Buddha, for two to three years and it did not help her. So she stopped practicing Buddhism.

Therapist's interpretations

The vast sand with just a small breathing oasis shows the severe and alarming depression of the client. The mother–child unity represented by the Native American mother holding a baby may be a good sign despite Jade's attempt to bury the figure. Of course, the upright piece of cedar wood is a protective figure. This piece was purchased at a local (Taiwanese) flower market. As I bought it, I was told that, in Asia, cedar wood represents a power that can dispel evils.

In the verbal portion of the session, Jade asked me what I would do if I were in her terrible condition. I replied that since I am a Christian, I would probably just pray to God and ask for His mercy. She asked more about my faith and indicated a desire to explore Christianity. I shared some Christian connections (names of pastors and churches) with her and told her that I would pray for her on a regular basis. I'd like to point out that when my clients are in serious troublesome conditions, as a practice, during my regular devotion, I would pray for them. This is helpful to me in that it gives me comfort and confidence. I also believe that my prayers are beneficial for the clients, too.

Sand picture 5

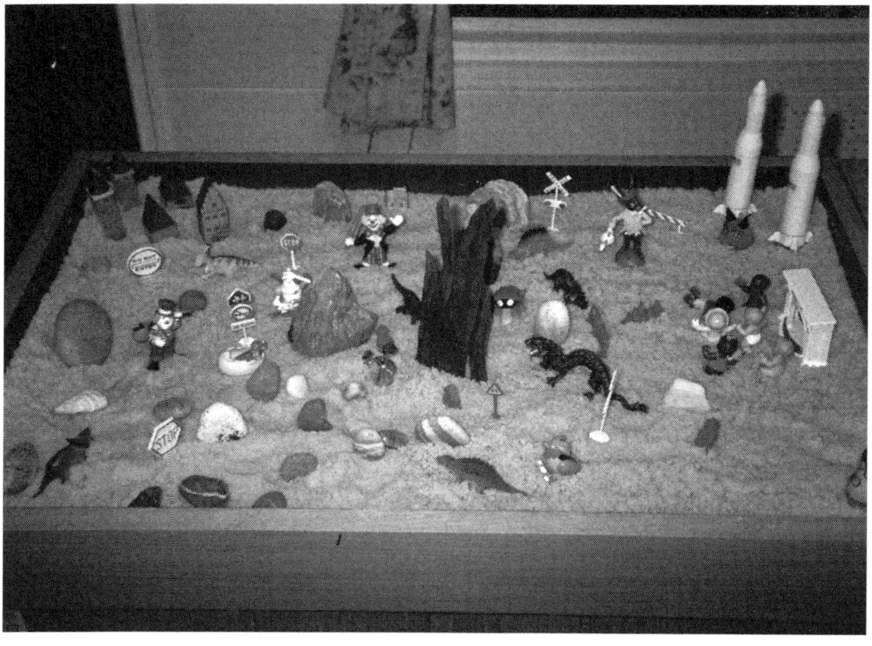

Figure 14.5 Fantasy world.

For the next several sessions, we continued to work on her depression. She did not like to do sand trays. Three months later, however, she came in and declared she wanted to do a tray.

Sand tray making process

Similar to the last few trays, she chose the wet tray. In contrast to the previous tray that contained just two items (Figure 14.4), she placed many items in this tray (Figure 14.5). In the upper left corner, there were several small wooden houses, whereas in the right upper corner, there were two rockets and a ghost mask (a red faced ghost with two black horns) sitting in front of the rockets. In the center of the right side, six babies were playing in front of a fireplace. A Russian nesting doll sat in the lower right corner.

At the very center of the tray, the cedar wood was again erected, surrounded by many items, especially a golden vase with roses that sat in front of the cedar wood. Other items were small stones and large upright stones, two clowns, many standing road signs, several dinosaurs, a dragon, a baby alligator breaking through its shell, and several fantasy figures.

Jade's comments

Upon finishing the tray, Jade crouched in front of the tray, looked at it closely, and commented:

> It is as if I am here, and I would really like to join them. In here, nobody controls anybody; there are no real people, and it is safer this way. The flowers [roses] are very powerful; they can dispel the danger . . . I really belong in this world. I am fit to be with them . . . Great! I am in touch with myself. This is what I want.

Therapist's interpretations

This tray differs a great deal from the previous tray. Jade's energy is highly elevated, reflected by the presence of two rockets, many playing children, the fireplace, the baby alligator emerging from its shell, and the deeper instinctual power as represented by dinosaurs and a dragon. The power of protection is shown again by the centering cedar wood and the "powerful" flowers as noted by Jade.

Clowns, two of them, under the protection of the masks, can act freely. Their white faces, though, may symbolize death. The cross design on their mouths suggests that they may be laughing at death. They can act, poke fun at themselves, and know how to fall and how to rise. Perhaps they are reflecting Jade's rising ability to laugh and joke at her past traumas, and her capacity to accept the alienated emotional self?

150 Author's sandplay case done in Taiwan

Many road signs are in this picture, including Stop, Do Not Enter, and Crossing signs. The Stop and Do Not Enter are protective signals, perhaps reflecting Jade's way of warning people not to harm her again. The Crossing sign may be the part of her that is saying "I am at the crossroad, and where do I go from here?"

Roses are known to be connected to a great goddess, a rebirth principle, and may represent the spring and youth (de Vries, 1984, p. 391). This concurred with Jade saying that they provide the source of power for her. In a retrospective review of the sand pictures, Jade said that in this sand picture, she feels she could breathe easily—she does not need a respirator (referring to the breathing hole that she made in the previous picture) any more.

Sand picture 6

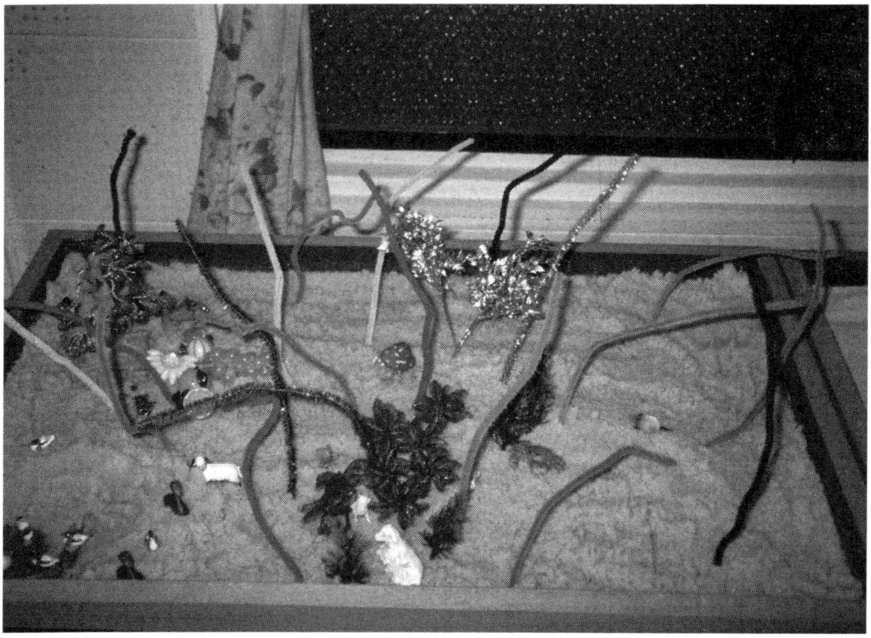

Figure 14.6 Fireworks of life.

Sand tray making process

Two weeks later, Jade made this sand picture (Figure 14.6). After placing many colorful pipe cleaners around the outer part of the tray, she began to place and to remove several fencing items (to make a fence) around the edge of the tray. These were: standing bricks, opened umbrellas, masks, and various small creatures. She decided not to use the fencing items. She kept two crabs (one cartoon figure), two mice (one cartoon figure), a snail, and a paper crane in the tray.

In the upper left corner sat a jewel tree and a variety of fruits plus carrots, whereas in the upper middle, golden branches lay. Lambs and a group of small ducklings plus two copper ducklings were either facing, nearby, or in the small lake that Jade made in the lower left corner. Small green trees were placed in the middle and lower middle of the tray.

Jade's comments

Jade noted that she had removed all items that made her uncomfortable and added that the pipe cleaners were more like her, not easy to control, and could go in different directions. She said that she really liked them. Then, she shared some family of origin issues, talking about frequent punishments that were administered to her by family members, as well as of her feeling of not belonging and not being wanted.

Therapist's interpretations

Many items in this tray, including discarding items, had never been selected by her in the past. The use of new items suggests that Jade is more at ease with trying something different and has more courage for the dangerous inner journey. Jade noted that, in retrospect, the pipe cleaners represented her courage and willingness to embark on a new adventure; they made her feel safe and she no longer had any need to avoid others. In my view, these colorful and freely-moving pipe cleaners represent the fireworks of her life and are ready to ignite it. Moreover, she chose to place food items that represent resources in the tray so they would be available for her use on her journey.

Sand picture 7

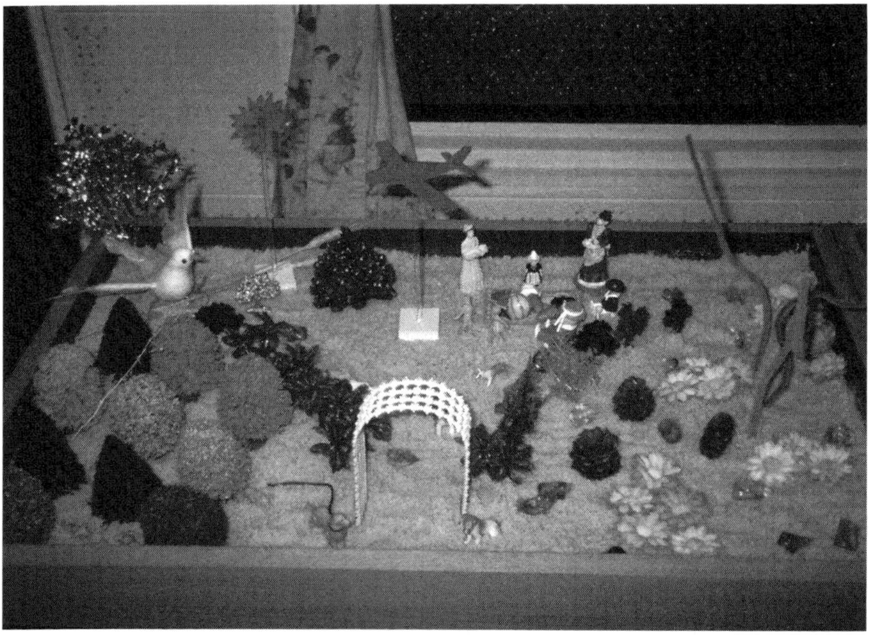

Figure 14.7 The gate.

Sand tray making process

Two weeks later, Jade made this tray (Figure 14.7). Behind the gate that is guarded by two dogs, there is a yard surrounded by two rows of trees. In a yard that had an airplane flying over it and a sun shining above it, there was a group of people (four children, a mother holding a baby, a woman holding a tray, and a sitting woman) encircling an area filled with fruits and ice cream cones. A large white dove with outstretched wings stood in front of golden and silver branches in the upper left corner. In the same area, there was a small golden tree and a tree full of jewels. More trees, flowers, glass rocks and colorful pipe cleaners were scattered around the tray, as were some animals, including little pigs running wild in the lower left corner.

Jade's comments

Upon completion of this tray, Jade crouched down and looked at it from the level of the tray. She seemed very pleased with this tray and said: "I like these shiny items. It is safe to place people in there. They seem lovable and happy. The pipe cleaners symbolize freedom."

Therapist's interpretations

This is the first time Jade put in a gate. It suggests that she has found an entrance to her inner world as well as to an outer peaceful world. The world that is inside the gate seems peaceful and pleasant as the children have mothers, friends, and food. This freedom is further mirrored by the flying airplane, the ready-to-fly dove, and the animals that are running free.

Sand picture 8

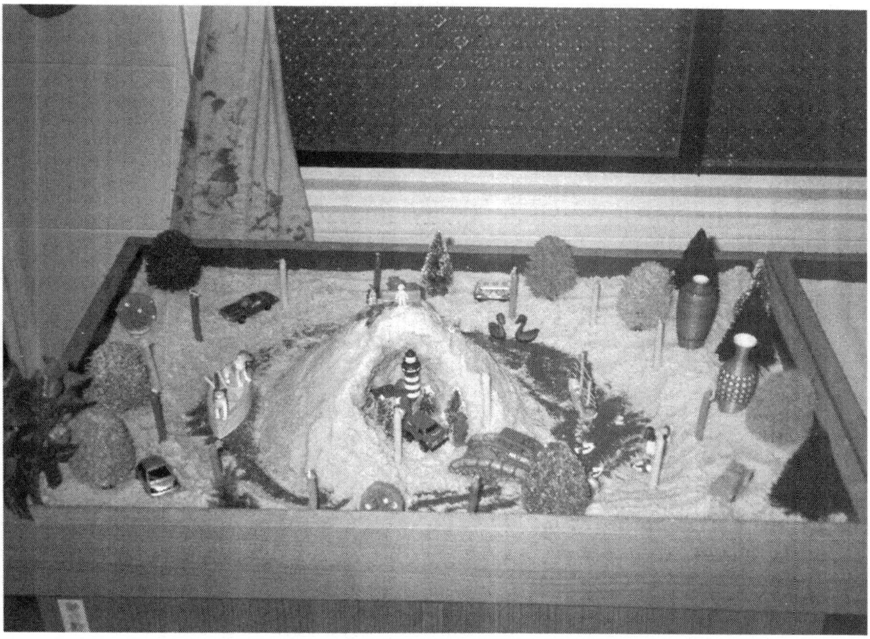

Figure 14.8 The safe hideout.

Three months later, Jade made this tray (Figure 14.8). In between the two trays presented in Figure 14.7 and Figure 14.8, she made three other trays. In those three trays, the same gate was present in two of them, one of them leading to a womb-like lake and two ships ready for use.

Sand tray making process

In the beginning, Jade carefully built a central mountain with a moat around it. In the center of this mountain, she dug out the sand and made a hideout with two candles standing in front of it, a lighthouse, four trees, and two people inside the mountain. A jeep was placed in the entrance, facing out, ready to take off. A bridge was placed on the moat, connecting the hideout to the outer world, and another vehicle was moving on the bridge. At the outer edge of the moat, a circle of candles were standing, and at the further outside edge, a circle of trees had been planted. Four additional vehicles were moving in the outer circle. In the moat, there was a sailboat and a rowboat with a dog and cat riding in it. A mother duck and several ducklings were in the water near the bridge, playing. Two beautiful vases were located in the upper and middle right. Toward the end of making this tray, Jade placed a bench on top of the mountain and a little figure sitting on the bench. Two birds, a hummingbird and a paper crane, were nearby.

Jade's comments

Jade said:

> It is so comfortable to sit at the highest place, peaceful, refreshing, and one can think clearly about things. At the hideout, one can move around. If one does not like to stay in, then he or she can go out. However, it is somewhat conflicting and not easy to decide whether to stay in or to go out.

Therapist's interpretations

There is a centering feel to this beautiful scene. According to Estelle Weinrib, the centering theme often occurs during the second stage of the sandplay process (Weinrib, 2004, p. 84). In my view, when a client is centering, he or she is often able to reach inside and find the inner psyche resources. In this tray, Jade built an inner psychic fort, and yet, it is not isolated. There is a bridge to connect the inner and the outer worlds. Vehicles are available for transportation.

A person sitting on top of the mountain with two birds accompanying her suggests the ability to reach upward for the resources or the power from above. The beautiful vases on the side of the tray were new items for Jade. As it turned out, she chose them many times for future trays, signifying the capacity for containment and signifying companionship. Jade often puts pairs of items in her trays, perhaps as a reflection of her need to be one with herself or with others.

A circle of candles are standing around the moat, and a lighthouse is inside the fort, giving an impression that light and energy are abundant, ready to be used.

Sand picture 9

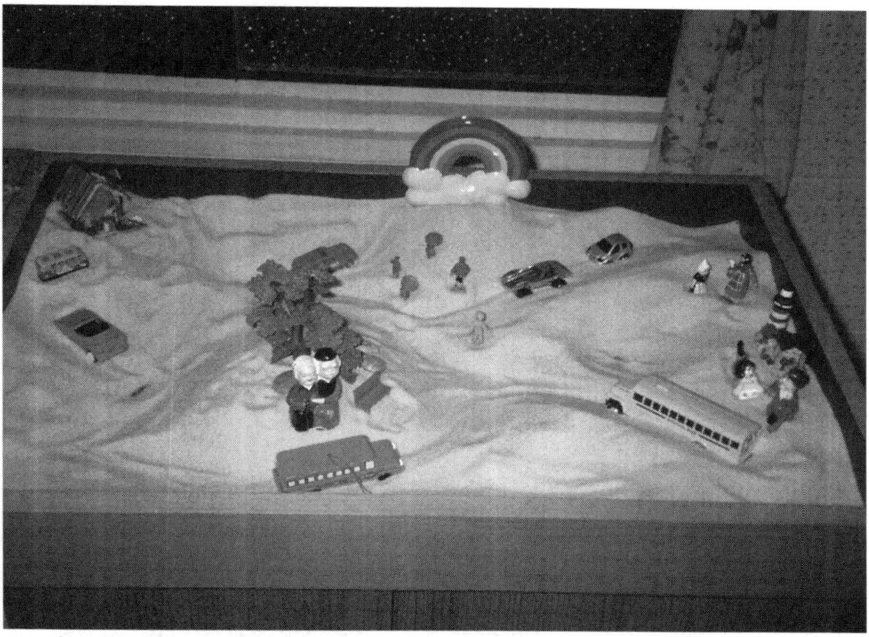

Figure 14.9 The flow in front of the rainbow.

This tray was made three months later (after a summer break that lasted three months). Before making the picture, Jade discussed her resistance to doing sand trays. She mentioned childhood experiences in which she had to please her mother by submitting to her mother's unrelenting needs. If she rebelled, her mother would lose control and threaten to commit suicide. Of interest, Jade made two sand trays this day.

Sand tray making process

Jade chose the dry sand to make the first tray (Figure 14.9). She caressed the sand slowly and steadily until it became the shape presented here. Then, she took sand and dribbled it through her fingers on to all surfaces. A huge rainbow and clouds were placed in the upper middle of the tray and in front of some hills. There were cars and school buses running around the trails that were built around the hills. A hut was placed in the upper left corner, whereas a lighthouse was located in the right middle. In the center toward the left side, an older couple (sitting) and a bench were placed under the oak tree. People were scattered in the hills and near the lighthouse.

Jade's comments

"Seeing the rainbow made me feel really great!" Jade said. She commented that there were no mountain climbers on the shelf, so she had to use other people to substitute for the climbers. She added that she put in many cars, and they were running.

Therapist's interpretations

After discussing her resistance, Jade chose the dry sand to do a tray. The way in which she was so intensely involved in making this tray was very moving to me. The rainbow, in Christianity, represents the covenant of peace that God promised to the people after the flood. Psychologically speaking, a severe depression seems like a huge flood that is so devastating. Perhaps the presence of the rainbow is a sign or a promise that there will be no more severe depression and no more suicidal ruminations.

Sand picture 10

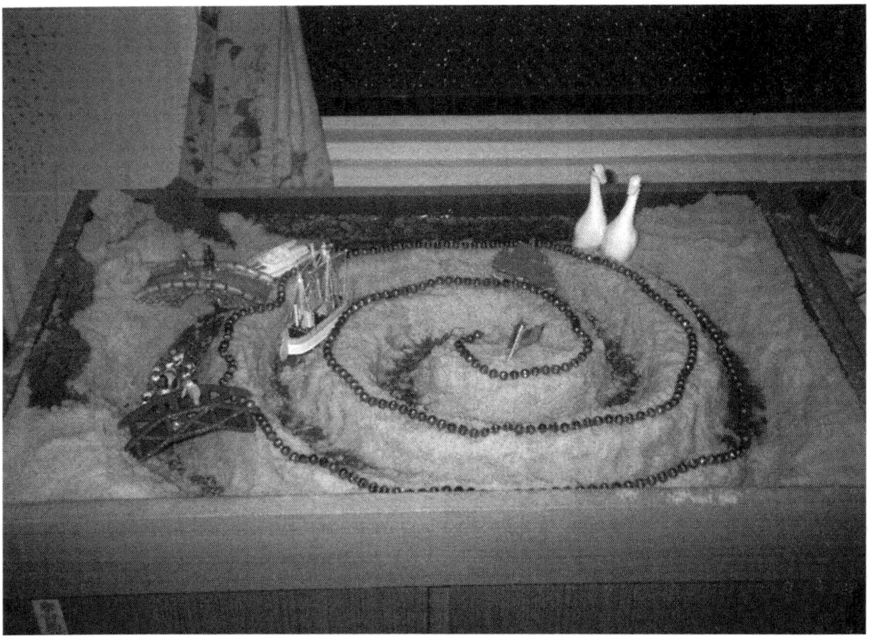

Figure 14.10 The spiral.

Sand tray making process

On the same day, using the wet sand, Jade spent a great deal of time making the spiral part of the sand (Figure 14.10). Then, she carefully placed a red beaded necklace on the top of the spiral. After that, she put in the following items: two flags (American and French) in the center, three boats, two huge white geese (upper right), two bridges (each has two persons walking on it, one toward the outer edge, one toward the center spiral), a mother duck and duckling (swimming in the water), and some sea reefs at the left outer land.

Jade's comments

Upon completion, Jade seemed relieved and said: "This spiral scene is really nice; it is flowing, moving very smoothly . . . I truly love the moving feel [of it]. I have found my voice. I have progressed, feeling good, and happy. I am very moved."

Therapist's interpretations

She was not the only one that was moved. I was very moved too. The spiral scene is very touching and beautiful. Besides, it is full of energy with the boats moving, people going in and out, and ducks swimming. At the time of this sand tray creation, the American and the French flags were the only flags that I had in the collection. Who knows what flags she might have used if I had other flags available? Regardless, the flags seem to reflect a centered target, the place to notice, to go to, and to protect.

Sand picture 11

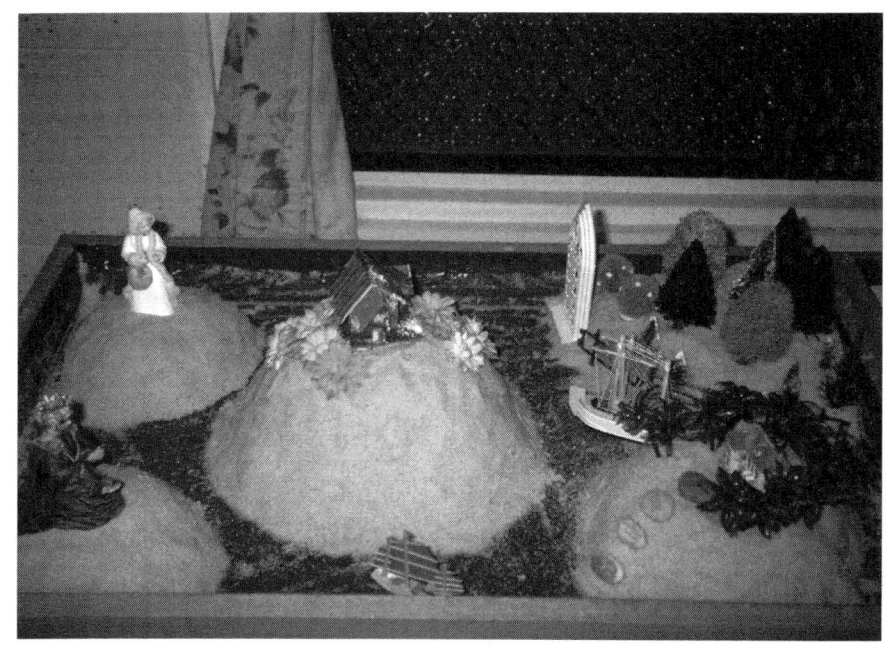

Figure 14.11 Five islands.

Sand tray making process

A month later, Jade crafted five islands with the center one somewhat bigger than the others (Figure 14.11). She put different items on each island. They were as follows: a straw house with flowers around it (center island); a woman carrying a flower basket (upper left island); a king wearing a crown (lower left island); a big white gate with trees behind it (upper right island); a house with trees around it and a stone path leading down to the water (lower right island). Three boats were present (one in the upper middle, not seen in this picture) and perhaps were moving around between islands.

Jade's comments

Jade said, "I like the center island; the house is located high ... There is distance between islands, so they won't be disturbed [by others] ... I like the feeling, smooth and free-flowing."

Therapist's interpretations

Jade expressed again her smooth and free-flowing feelings in this creation. Five islands could represent different parts of herself with the center island reflecting the maturing ego, whereas the woman and the king might represent the internalized mother and father images or the not-yet-integrated yin and yang principles. Boats are available to connect the islands. Thus, the hope for further integration is present.

In his book of which I read the Chinese translation (Chinen, 1999, pp. 38–39), Allan Chinen indicated that the number five is a characteristic of midlife. It is one more than the four that Jung regards as integration and wholeness. Thus, it symbolizes above or over, in a material or sensory sense. Chinen points out that five may represent wanting more and perhaps materialism, while de Vries (1984, p. 191) says that five has multiple symbolic meanings; it can represent progress, the power that will change nature, or the wisdom and the light that comes from above.

Since Jade is nearing her midlife age, the five here may suggest a possible midlife crisis. This is somewhat confirmed by the next sand picture, which is not shown in this text. She made another five lands in one tray with one land being a large graveyard and the center land (a lake) shaped like a huge coffin covered with many small items, including shiny buttons, little bells, and a glass ball. The graveyard and the coffin-shaped lake suggest the possible recurrence of depression.

Sand picture 12

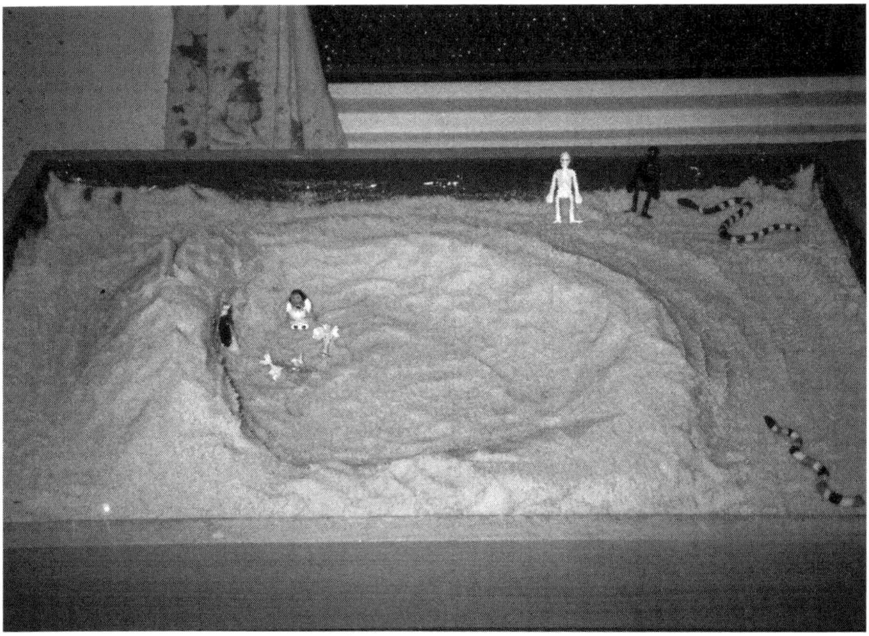

Figure 14.12 A solid fort.

Jade made two more trays (including the aforementioned five lands with the centered coffin-shaped lake) before this tray, which was made three months after the last shown sand picture (Figure 14.11).

Sand tray making process

At the beginning of this session, Jade struggled a lot about whether she would or would not do a tray. She finally decided to give it a try (Figure 14.12). First, she put a witch in the wet sand. Then she piled up some sand and moved the witch to the top of the mound. Jade seemed uncomfortable and replaced the witch with a cross. Then she put a priest on the right side of the sand pile and proceeded to craft the sand pile into a solid, round-shaped fort. Using two wood sticks, she transported two large snakes into the tray, one in the upper right corner and another in the lower right corner. Then she placed two skeletons, one white and one black near the snake in the upper right corner. The last items she put in the tray were the little native girl with a drum in front of her and some flowers.

Jade's comments

Upon finishing the tray, Jade said:

> After placing the snakes, my stomach hurt a lot. Moreover, the witch wasn't what I wanted. Was I sick? I really did not know what I wanted. But then I found the cross and put it in. After that, I felt powerful, hopeful, and safe. The little girl could finally come out. When I could not find myself, I felt like I might as well kill myself.

Therapist's interpretations

The tray and her comments say it all. Jade had been depressed and perhaps suicidal again. She said she was sad because nobody remembered her birthday that was a few days ago, and it just went by. In addition, her work was rather stressful. I would like to note that Jade is very fearful of snakes; she did not dare to touch them so she used sticks to pick them up. Hopeful signs: she did put snakes in the tray, no matter how she accomplished the feat; she built a solid fort, and she used the cross image to comfort herself.

Sand picture 13

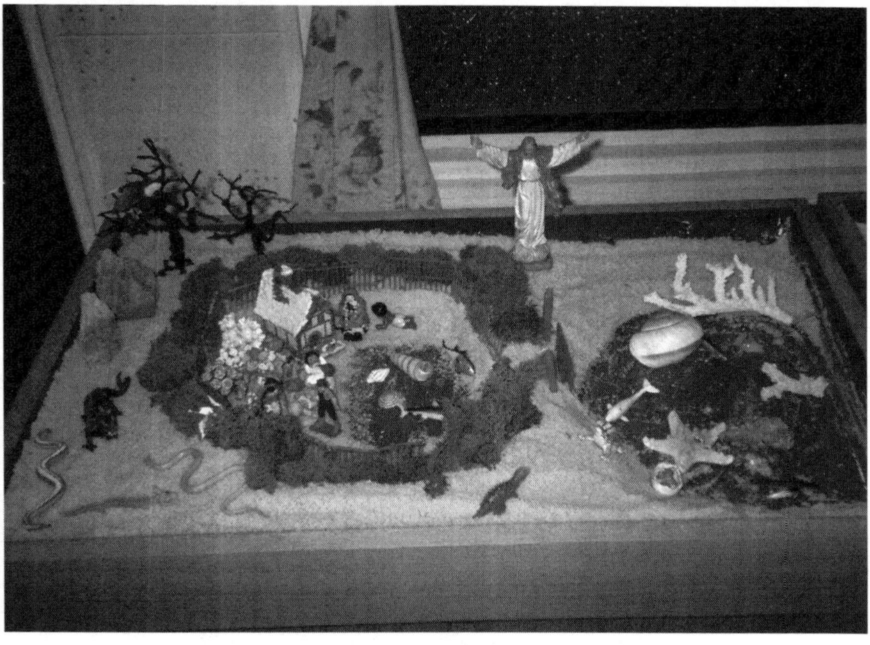

Figure 14.13 After all, I am not an unwanted child!

Jade made two more trays between the previously shown sand picture and this one (Figure 14.13). The first one was similar to the previous one (Figure 14.12). She made another very solid fort with a cross standing on it, and a little baby and a priest were inside the fort. No snakes and no skeletons were present. Jade is represented by the baby figure, who is frightened, and yet protected (by a priest and a cross), with the threatening figures gone. In the next tray, she placed a pair of praying hands in the middle of the right side and many new items in the left side of the tray—including many babies, some aboriginal people, a family of giraffes, fishes, and a huge starfish. Upon completion, Jade said that she felt safe and that it was good to be in touch with the primitive figures.

Sand tray making process

This tray was made two months after Figure 14.12. In the wet tray, Jade dug out two lakes with the one on the right being somewhat larger than the one on the left, and they had a tunnel connecting them. After placing fences and trees (surrounding the left lake) on the left side of the tray, she built a home near the left lake and an entrance for the left homeland. Inside the homeland, she placed a house with flowers on the side, children and babies playing, working adults, and a storyteller. There was a baby crawling toward the storyteller. There were fishes and shells in the lake. On the shore of the right-hand lake, there were also fishes, a big shell, a large starfish, some coral stones, an alligator, and a baby alligator breaking through its shell.

In the upper left corner of the tray, there were two dried trees. An eagle was sitting on top of one tree. Beneath the dead tress, there were two stone-made mountains. In the lower left area, there were two snakes and two dragons. A small dinosaur was placed in the lower middle. Finally, in the upper middle area, Jade placed a huge Christian figure—Jesus holding his hands up high.

Jade's comments

After completing the tray, Jade said, "I feel very happy! I love ocean waves, and I have less fear of the water. I miss my father very much" (note: he passed away years ago). After some discussion about her father, she concluded that her father, though often remaining silent, made her feel that, "After all, I am not an unwanted child."

Therapist's interpretations

The significant difference between this home and the home in the first sand tray (Figure 14.1) is the fact that there is interaction between the children and the adults in this tray. A black baby is crawling toward a Native American storyteller who represents love for the children, cultural inheritance, and tradition. In spite of several threatening figures, e.g., snakes, alligator, dragons, appearing in the outer world, the upheld hands of the large figurine of Jesus seem to signify a strong protective power. The connection between the two sides by a tunnel is of interest. Jade seems less split, more willing to integrate her two sides. Jade had started to attend some church activities and felt somewhat helped by church members.

Sand picture 14

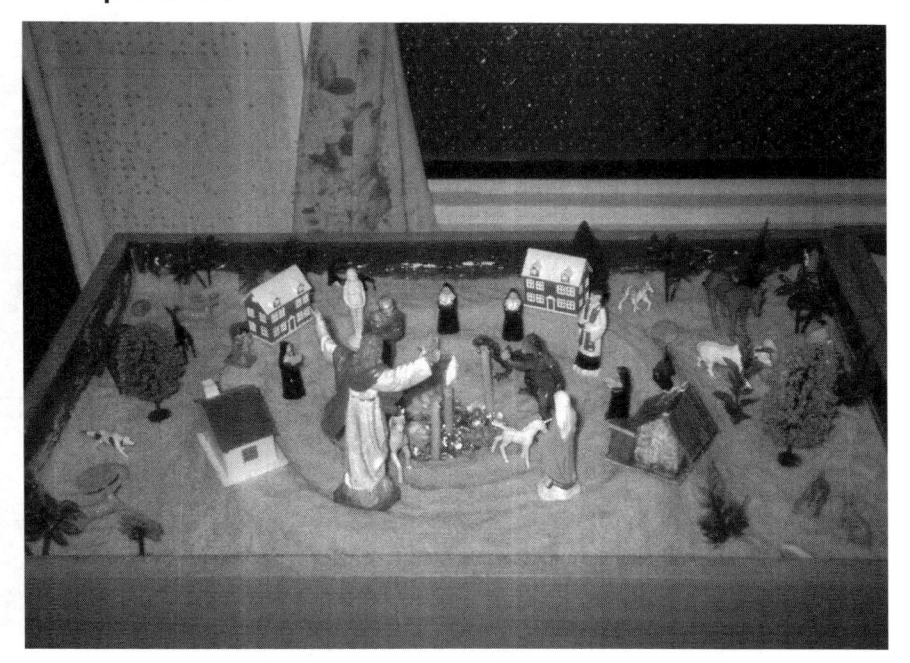

Figure 14.14 Mandala.

Sand tray making process

Two-and-a-half months and three more sand trays later, Jade made this tray (Figure 14.14). She intensely and laboriously crafted the center part of the tray. There was a center circle which was a pond decorated with glass marbles, three flowers, and five candles—it was the lowest in elevation. The three surrounding circles were made of sand, very rounded, very firmly packed, centered, and each outer circle was slightly more elevated than the previous one.

In the first circle located near the center of the tray, Jade placed one dragon, three unicorns, and a Neanderthal couple with the female holding a baby. In the second circle, she placed four nuns, a pregnant woman, a priest, the Virgin Mary, and Jesus, the one who is holding up his hands. In the third, she put four houses and two Native American mothers holding babies. In the outer area of this mandala creation, there were several animals, including many horses, deer, and goats, as well as trees and stones. At the end, Jade lit one candle, the one in the center.

Jade's comments

Jade said that the shape of the circle had frequently been on her mind lately. Today she made a decision to use it. She also felt that in the center there must be a lit candle. She added:

> At the beginning, I worried that I was incapable of making it. However, I decided to give it a try, and I am very happy that I completed it. I feel so at ease now, very moved, a bit bittersweet, and numinous. Moreover, I feel very safe and very relieved that I have arrived at the center.

Therapist's interpretations

During the time Jade was diligently making these layers of circle creation, I felt very moved and thought that it was sacred. It is well known in the sandplay community that when both the therapist and the client are moved or touched by a sand tray, it is likely that a Self Tray has been created. Dora Kalff (2003, p. 5), the founder of sandplay, termed it "the manifestation of Self." This circling phenomenon may also be called a "mandala" that is characterized by feelings of holiness, integrity, and beauty when it occurs.

In this tray, the number four, which is regarded as representing wholeness and integrity, is shown in many places: four circles, four houses, four nuns, and four horses. Perhaps, as Jade said, she has reached the center of the psyche; therefore the possibility of becoming whole and integrated is not far away. The client's life, resembling the burning candle, is starting to shine.

Sand picture 15

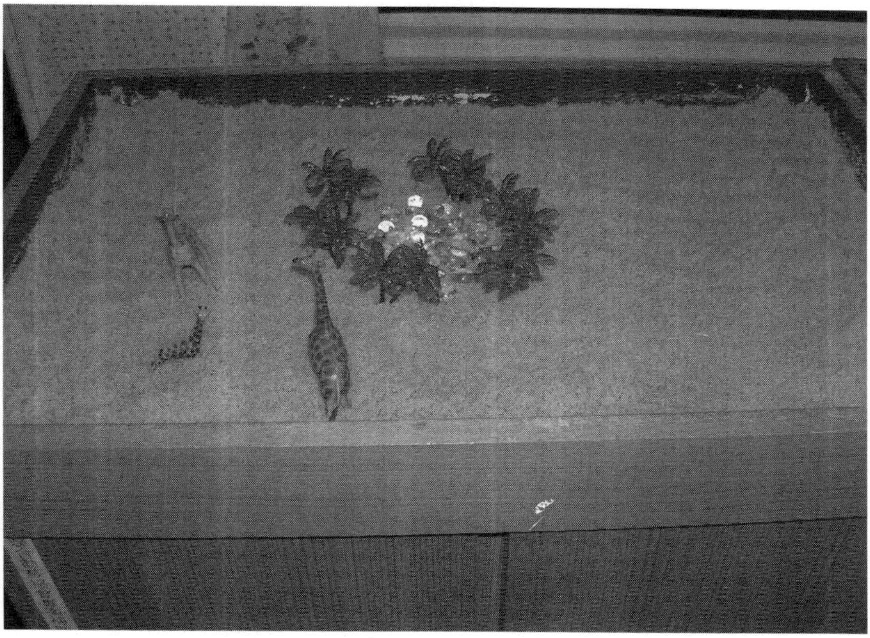

Figure 14.15 Tears.

Two more very beautiful mandala scenes were crafted by Jade after Figure 14.14. Jade seemed to enjoy these creations very much. Then came a summer break of two and a half months. The above sand picture (Figure 14.15) was made right after the break.

Sand tray making process

At the onset of the session, Jade seemed very tense and anxious as she said, "I do not like the feeling of not finding myself!" She thought of making a tray, but she did not know what to make. She then noted that she wanted to make a "perfect" tray, and she was very uneasy.

When asked whether she was angry at the therapist for taking a break, she vehemently rejected the notion and proceeded to make a tray. During the entire process of tray making, she was in tears. At first, she loudly and tearfully announced, "I want to put trees in!" and she did. Then, she said, "I do not want colorful marbles" and chose only the transparent marbles, placed them in the center, and said, "These are what I want!!" Then she loudly stated, "I want to put some animals in!" She chose three giraffes (this is the sixth time she has placed the giraffe family in the tray), put them in and said, "I am done!"

During the making of this tray, I told her repeatedly, "Feel free to do whatever you want or to place anything you want!"

Jade's comments

Upon completion, Jade seemed to awake from a bad dream. She said, "I have fought a huge war!"

Therapist's interpretations

Indeed, Jade fought a big war, and she won. After denying any negative transference, she entered a war within herself through the sand tray making. The positive encouragement from the therapist appeared to have relieved her from her anxiety about harboring anger toward the therapist. Furthermore, Jade's insistence on placing certain items in the tray and being firm about not putting in anything she did not want seemed to calm her down.

In this session, Jade went from "I do not know what I want" to "I found myself, and I know what I want!" The transparent marbles in the center of the tray, resembling the tears that were in her eyes throughout the entire sand tray making, seemed to be shining and cleansing.

Sand picture 16

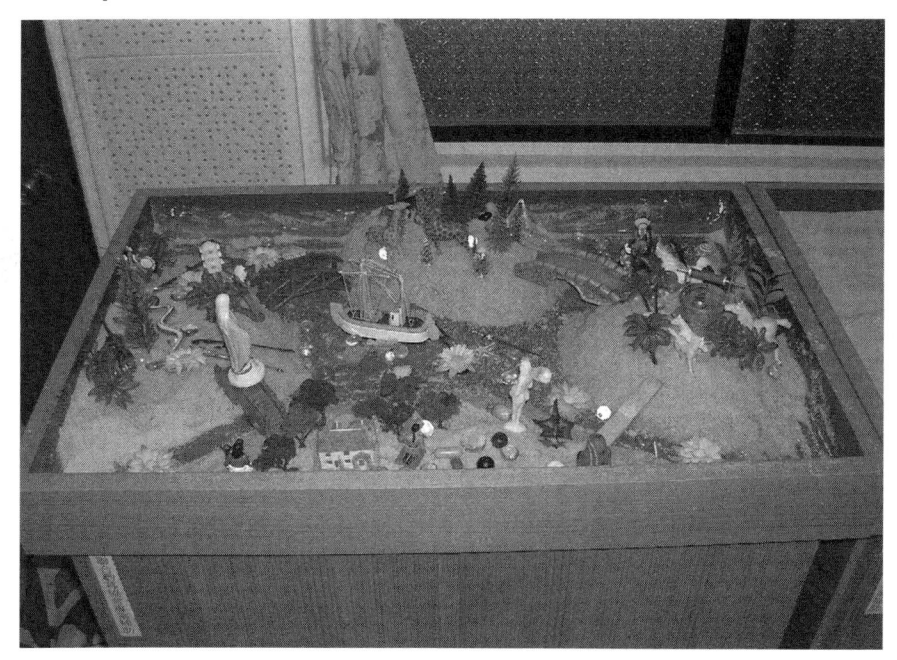

Figure 14.16 Four connecting islands.

After making two highly-centered sand scenes that were full of energy, resource, and blessing, Jade made this tray (Figure 14.16) about one-and-a-half months after the previously shown sand picture.

Sand tray making process

Jade crafted an island in the upper center, and then she molded and made three other islands. On the upper centered island, she placed trees, fruits, and the giraffe family. On the left centered island, she put trees, flowers, two Native American figures (a drummer and a chief), a large snake, and a fierce tiger. There were swords on the island as well as in the water. A streetlight was put in last.

On the right center island, she placed a well and its little bucket, trees, and a unicorn family of four. On the island located in the lower center, there were trees, fruits, three mothers holding babies, a pregnant woman, and a storyteller. Marbles of different colors and flowers were scattered all over the tray—either on the islands or in the water. Four bridges and two boats, including a canoe (upper right) that carried a Native American chief and another Native American male, were present. At the very last moment, Jade put a Virgin Mary figure on top of one bridge (lower left).

Jade's comments

Jade said she felt powerful because she dared to put in a large snake (she used sticks to place it) and the swords. She noted that the lower island was the land for breeding, whereas the upper island contained peaceful feelings. She felt the whole tray was numinous and mysterious. However, she noted that in order to make it safe for the giraffe family, she had to put in a streetlight as a warning (of the large snake) and swords to protect the family. She also indicated that the tiger and the Native Americans had protective powers, trying to keep the place safe. Lastly, she commented that the Virgin Mary was the most powerful of all—and a protector of everyone.

Therapist's interpretations

Jade previously created a five-island (unconnected) scene, whereas here, she made a four-island one, and they are connected by four bridges. Four, a dominant theme here, is commonly known by Jungians as representing wholeness, perfection, and integrity. Chinen (1999, p. 38) pointed out that the number four may represent the searching for wholeness and integrity by older people. Although Jade is not yet in that age demographic, her tray here shows the power, strength, and wholeness that she is developing.

An attempt at a union of opposites is clearly shown in the yang power of the left center island and the yin elements of the connecting lower center island, plus the yang strength of the upper right (the canoe with two male Native Americans) and the yin protective power of the Virgin Mary in the lower left. The yin and yang elements are either connected by a bridge, or interacting at opposite ends of each other.

Sand picture 17

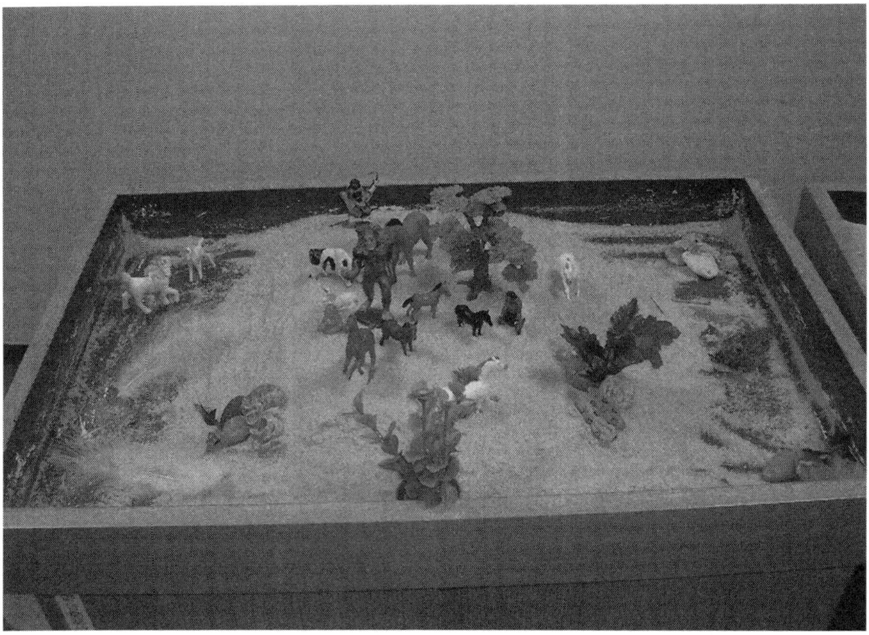

Figure 14.17 The lonely island.

Jade made three more trays in the two months between the previous session and this one. Those three trays were "Abundant nurturing," "Extraordinarily beautiful world," and "Celebration" as I named them.

Sand tray making process

Jade pushed the sand from both sides of the tray into the middle and formed a large island with a flat top (Figure 14.17). On this island, she placed several horses, trees and flowers, a cow, a small unicorn, and two snakes (she still used sticks to grab them) by some stones. There were also Native Americans, a Neanderthal, an archer, and a small birthing woman. In the four corners were: two frogs on stones (upper right); two unicorns (upper left); two stones and a leaf (lower right); and two feathers (lower left).

Jade's comments

Upon completion, Jade said: "Snakes are very fearsome and disgusting! Arranging horses and people in the upper ground and snakes in the lower location makes it safer." She further commented that moving here (the therapy place had been moved to another location) is good because there is more room. However, she said it is more difficult to find figurines and the newness makes her somewhat uncomfortable.

Therapist's interpretations

In contrast to the previous three trays, Jade placed considerably fewer items in this tray. The moving of the therapy venue seemed to have disturbed her considerably. She made a lonely island ground with significantly threatening snake figures at the bottom and fewer resources and protective power. The pairs in this tray again seem to reflect her splitting selves—loneliness and a need for companionship.

Sand picture 18

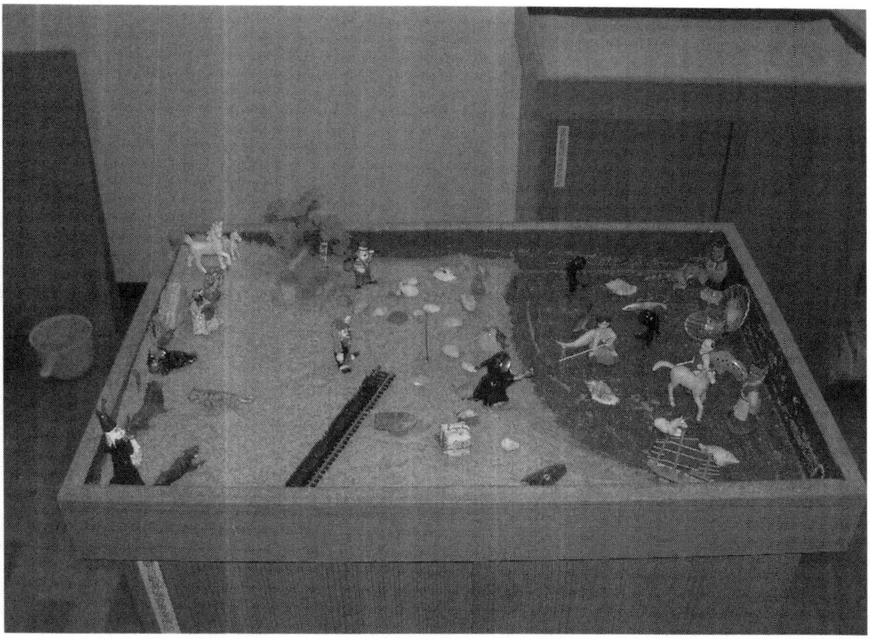

Figure 14.18 Sea and land.

Sand tray making process

Four weeks later, Jade made this tray (Figure 14.18). This was a sea and land with a hill scene. There were many items in both areas. In the sea, there were: many fishes; two opened shells that contained marbles; several Asian gods and goddesses; a sailboat; two unicorns; and shells. In the land with a hill area, there were: many shells and stones; several masks; a witch; a heart-shaped metal (that is rusted) figure that was upright; a gift package; and a cartoon bear grabbing a fish in its paw along the shore line. In the mid to lower center, a train was placed on the track, perhaps moving. In the upper middle and the center of the tray, there were clowns. A Japanese-style house for travelers and an oak tree were near the upper clown. In the outer right area, these items (from top to bottom) were placed: two unicorns; a mask; a small glass snake (Jade used her hand to grab this snake); an owl; an Asian male with a musical instrument and a hummingbird (the above three items are near an upright stone); another Asian male; a small moon figure; three fierce animals (a lion king, a leopard, and a tiger); and a Merlin figurine who is holding a fire and a cane.

Jade's comments

At completion of the tray, Jade said, "The gods and goddesses in the water are powerful. They can go up the mountain and can go down to the sea." She added that the witch can fly, though. Jade said she likes the water side because it is firmer and more real, whereas if one is on the upper right hill, one can be lonely. She noted that she is a bit confused and could not understand her feelings. She also commented that her creativity is at its highest and that it makes her feel really good.

Therapist's interpretations

Jade somewhat impulsively and yet a bit compulsively put many items in the tray. The opposing or splitting selves are depicted by the clear division of the land and the sea, and the Asian goddess and the Western witch with the two of them facing and opposing each other. Many masks and two clowns appear to be disdainfully observing the funny and contradictory world. The rusted heart in the center (not seen in this picture), however, suggests a possibility for transformation. Also, this is the first time that Jade dared to grab a snake by hand and put it in the tray.

In this very active (many things are moving) and yet somewhat confusing tray, I sensed Jade's splitting manic-depressive trait. When a client is reaching the Self part, they can be very high, creative, and sometimes manic. Steps must be taken to release the high energy at times while protecting the self. Jade chose to do many projects at home and this provided her a chance to release the abundant and somewhat out-of-control energy.

Sand picture 19

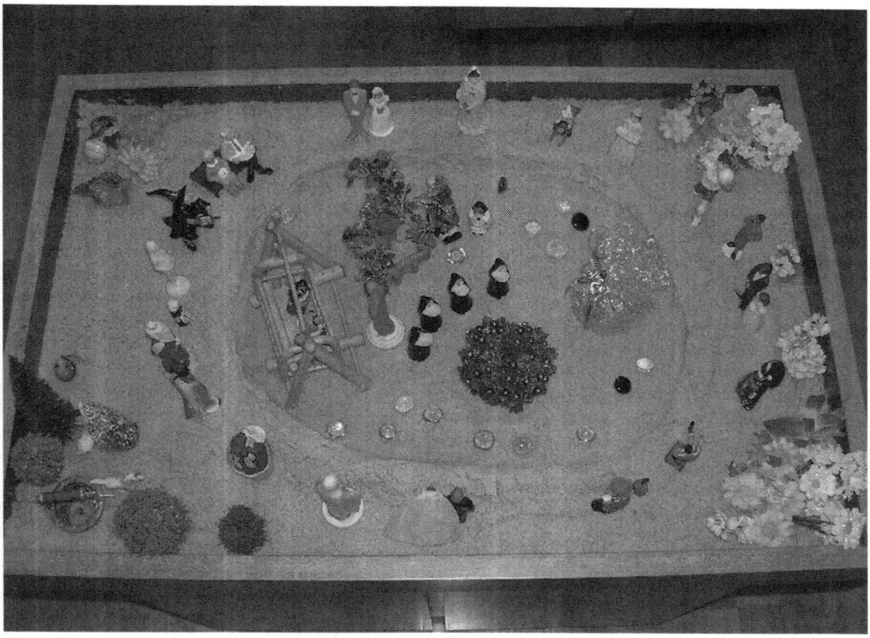

Figure 14.19 Reappearance of mandala.

Sand tray making process

Upon arriving for this session, Jade proceeded to give me a gift—an arty notebook, a project that she had completed. She appeared proud. Then, she immediately went to work on a sand tray (Figure 14.19). She carefully and diligently crafted a huge, indented circle in the middle part of the tray. Outside the circle, she placed the following items: Guan Yin; a little boy riding a sled; a mother holding a baby; a girl playing volleyball; a teenage black boy on the phone; a newlywed couple; an Asian girl; a soccer player; a clown; another newlywed couple; the Virgin Mary; a woman holding a tray; a standing Asian male (one of the seven wise men); an Asian god; a little girl; a pregnant woman; a witch; a sitting older couple; and another wedding couple.

Inside the circle, she placed the following items: a huge bamboo cradle with two little Asian girls; two Virgin Mary figurines overlooking the cradle; four nuns; a storyteller; a little Native American girl with a drum; a jewel tree; a Christmas tree; a glass ball with a gold-colored wrapper; and some marbles. In the very outer area, she placed: fruits (upper left); flowers (upper right and lower right); trees; two unicorns; a well; and the glass snake (lower left). Again, Jade used her hand to place the snake in the tray.

Jade's comments

She said, "I feel very good and right. I like this area [pointing to the center area] very much. It is very centering, very together."

Therapist's interpretations

After making a splitting or fighting (between two sides) tray (Figure 14.18), Jade made this beautiful, orderly, and centering tray. This is the reappearance of a mandala, or a Self tray. Without any doubt, she has reached that precious psyche center again. Perhaps this centering will help her to be more stable?

Also, this is the first time that she has placed a cradle in the tray. In this safe container, there are two little girls protected by the Virgin Mary. Within the outer big container, there is also the girl with a drum near the storyteller who has many children in her arms. The presence of a protective theme reinforces the psychological strength that Jade has built for herself.

Moreover, the placement of many newlywed couples plus the older couple, and the presence of a witch and a wise man, the Guan Yin of Buddhism, and the Virgin Mary of Christian religion, all point to the union of opposites that is so crucial in the development of a healthy psyche. The recurrence of the four singing nuns is of significance. Nuns remain single; they do not rely on men. They signify the independence and inner wholeness that Jade has been trying to obtain.

Sand picture 20

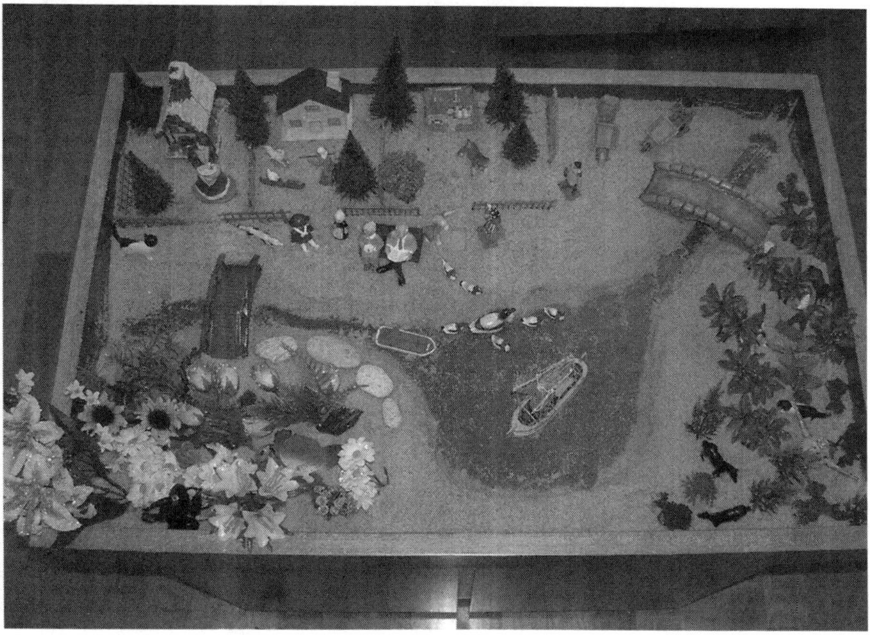

Figure 14.20 Peaceful homeland.

Sand tray making process

Jade divided the sand into three areas (top, lower left and lower right) with a middle lake and a waterway that extended into both sides (Figure 14.20). There were two bridges; they connect the upper land with the two lower lands. Two boats were on the lake. Near the upper lake shore, a duck family casually swam. In the upper big land, there was a village scene where children, parents, working adults, and older people resided. Domestic animals were present and also freely roamed between the upper and lower right lands. There was a working male adult in the lower right land as well. In the lower left land, there was a witch and a glass-made snake that Jade bravely grabbed and placed. The snake was partially hidden under the huge piles of flowers and plants.

Jade's comments

Upon arriving at this session that was held two weeks after the previous one, Jade said that she had been preoccupied with the round-shaped theme and wanted to change it. Although somewhat reluctant, she proceeded to make a homeland in the upper area that was not characterized by roundness. Upon completion, she noted that she felt solid, grounded, and normal. She further commented that since she gave me a gift of her creation last session, she felt more at ease, more stable, and not as manic.

Therapist's interpretations

Jade used creative activities to deal with her tremendously flowing and manic energy and eventually began to stabilize. Significantly, she became even more stable after giving me a gift that she had made by hand. This giving and receiving can be viewed as a type of co-transference that brings about a stabilizing force for the client.

In this beautiful and peaceful homeland that Jade created, people and animals are free to do as they please. The working adults, the resting older couple, and the playing children, accompanied by their pets, all seem to be living comfortably; it is truly a peaceful scene.

Interestingly, in the lower left area where Jade used to have a graveyard and flowers, the flowers are still there. However, the graves and gravestones are gone. In their place are a witch and a snake. Although they may be viewed as frightening and evil, the witch and the snake are known for having transforming powers and can be healing. In addition, an owl with outstretched wings in the lower right may signify the increasing psychological wisdom that can help Jade to face future challenges.

Sand picture 21

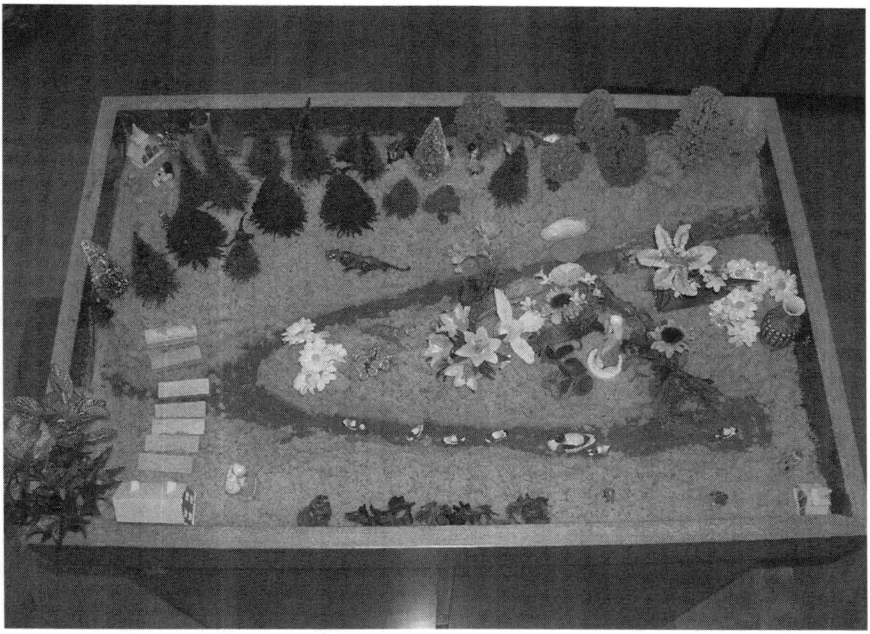

Figure 14.21 Almost home!

Sand tray making process

Two weeks later, Jade made this tray (Figure 14.21). As in the previous tray, she divided the sand into three areas that were separated by a stream and connected on the left side by a bridge made of wooden steps. Two small churches were placed, one in the upper left corner, one in the lower right corner, facing each other over a great distance. Near the center of the tray, Jade placed a white dove and a Virgin Mary figure. To their right was a standing vase.

In the upper left corner, Jade built a small village, whereas in the lower left corner, she placed a house with a mother holding a baby in front. Animals and fantasy animals roamed all over the tray, and the duck family was in the stream. Many trees were placed in the upper area, flowers were placed in the middle, and some dry flowers and a huge plant were located at the bottom.

Jade's comments

Jade stated that she had had a dream the previous night, and in the dream, she found herself located in a deep and faraway mountain area—thus, she made this scene. She noted that the little village in the mountain was where she belonged. In this mountain-village that she liked, tiger and leopard could freely go in and out, people and animals peacefully cohabited, and there was no danger. She added, "I am almost home!"

Therapist's interpretations

When Jade made this tray, she was very involved. She devoted a great deal of time to molding the sand and to choosing the items that she wanted to place in the tray, especially in the upper left area, which she said was her deep and faraway mountain home. This faraway place where people and fierce animals can peacefully live together reminds me of the Garden of Eden that was created by God and was a very perfect living place for all. It also suggests that Jade has reached the psyche center where an integration of her ego and shadow is likely taking place.

The presence of two churches facing each other over a far distance, the white dove and the Virgin Mary figurine, and the steps leading to the faraway mountain home all have a numinous quality, giving the scene an awesome feel.

Sand picture 22

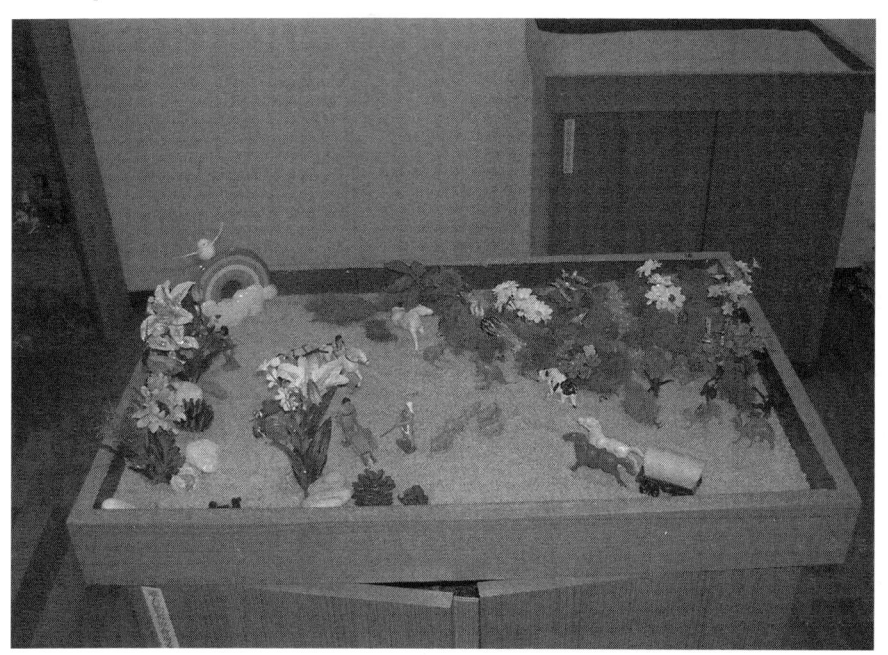

Figure 14.22 Going toward the light.

Before making this sand picture (Figure 14.22), Jade made three trays that were related to a blessed homeland where there were abundant life energy and love. We also dealt with her anxiety about termination. "I love sandplay so much, and I can't be separated from it," she said.

Sand tray making process

Jade placed a two-horse carriage in the lower right corner of the tray, and it was heading toward the upper left corner where a white dove rested on a rainbow above the clouds. A Native American woman on a horse located in the center/left headed toward the lower right. A pig family was walking across the road near the center of the road while many animals roamed in the upper right forest. Working adults and Native people were present all over the tray. In this tray, Jade placed new animals that she had not used in the past, including monkeys, kangaroos, and camels. She also placed a little green snake in the tray (near the butterfly) with her hand. She seemed more at ease in grabbing this snake.

Jade's comments

Jade said, "My heart feels just like the horse carriage. It is going toward a faraway place. It is an old and spiritual place, very far away. I will go toward it!"

Therapist's interpretations

Jade is maturing. She carries the power of the horse and the horse carriage. She seems ready to be on her own to continue with her journey. In this session, she told me that she is ready to say goodbye to her mother, who is in her eighties (if her mother wishes to go). When a client is near the end of the sandplay process, a going-away scene may show up, hinting the readiness of the client to end the process. Of significance, the placement of several new animals in this tray suggests Jade's expanding flexibility in terms of her instinctual power, resources, and expressions.

Sand picture 23

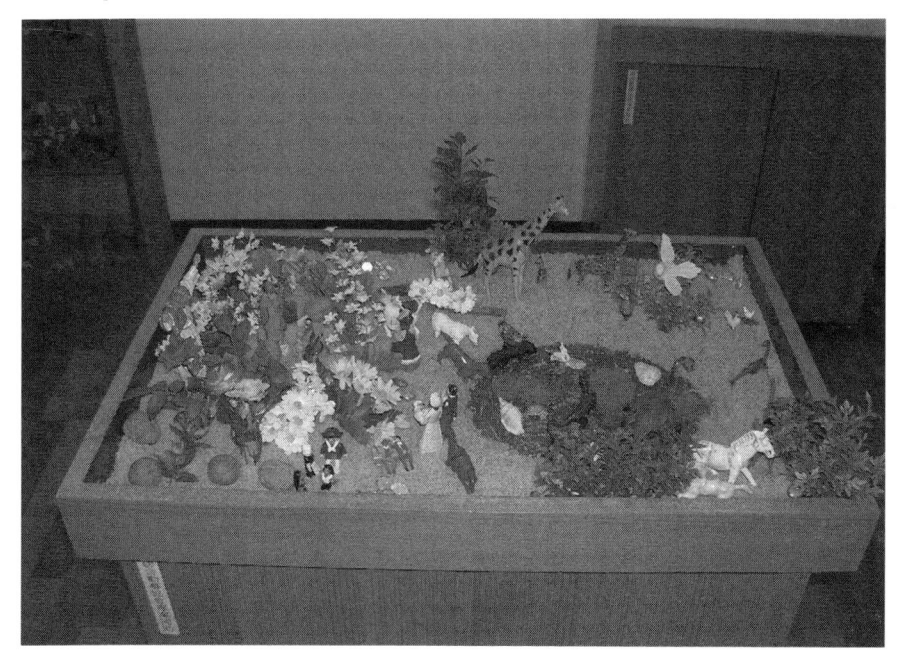

Figure 14.23 Deep and firm blessings.

Sand tray making process

Jade crafted a very rounded lake at the right side of the tray (Figure 14.23). In the lake, there were two dragons, a crane, shells, a piece of stone. There were two horses and a bird on a log on the shore. In the left center, she placed the Jesus figurine with upheld hands and then a Virgin Mary figurine. Then, in front of Jesus, Jade placed a nest with eggs and a mother bird.

In the garden on the left side of the tray, flowers bloomed and nuts were on the ground. Human figurines that were arranged in front of Jesus and Mary included a couple of children, two Japanese girls right at the foot of the Virgin Mary, a woman holding a tray near the center, and a couple with the mother holding a baby near lower center. Another group of children and two persons sitting on a bench were also present.

Animals and fantasy creatures were placed all over the tray, including horses, unicorns, a family of giraffes, a family of chickens, dinosaurs, and a white dove. At left of center, under the foot of the Virgin Mary and by the children, is the little green snake that Jade has been using. At the end of making this tray, Jade placed glass marbles in several locations.

Jade's comments

Upon completion of this tray, Jade said:

> The garden on the left side seems to be above the cloud; it feels like floating. Now I am feeling like an independent individual, a bit lonely, but I am maturing. I feel that my Christian faith has helped me a lot. It is a kind of trusting, and it gives me a feeling of permanence as well as stability. In this process, I have found myself, my family, and my home. I feel very stable, very clear and deep, a tiny bit sad, but very blessed.

Therapist's interpretations

This is, indeed, a beautiful garden, like the Garden of Eden, full of peace, energy, resources, love, and protection. The round, clear, deep lake seems to be a source of nurturance, providing a fountain of life for all. Not only is Jade feeling blessed, but also I who have witnessed such a deep and beautiful process am truly blessed.

Sand picture 24

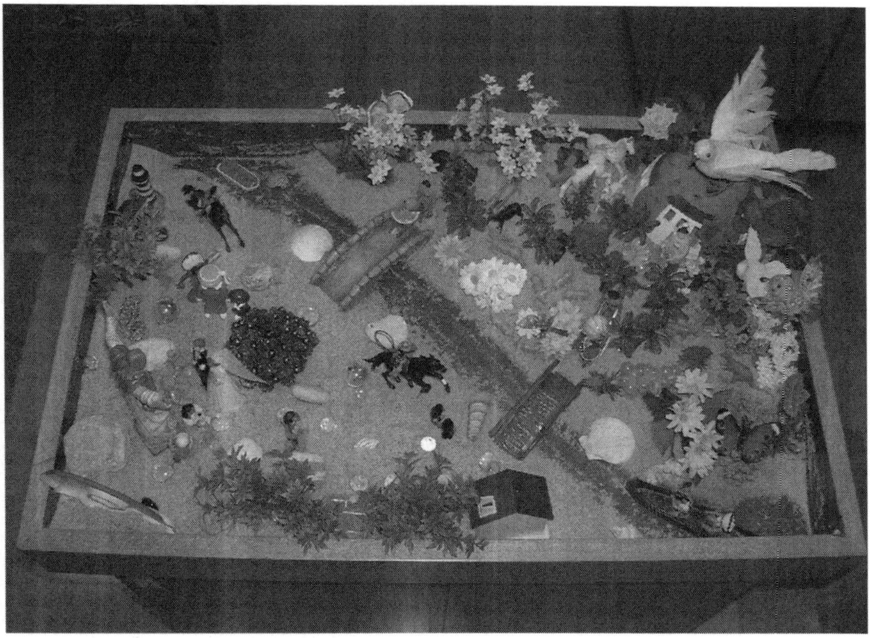

Figure 14.24 Rebirth.

Three weeks after the previous tray, Jade made another centered, peaceful, beautiful scene in which a feeling of being blessed is very evident. Two weeks later, she made this final tray (Figure 14.24).

Sand tray making process

Jade crafted a river that ran from the lower right to the upper left of the tray. This river divided the tray into two halves that were connected by two bridges. In the upper right corner, she placed a dome-shaped, colorful building and on top of it, a huge white resting dove with raised wings. A family of unicorns resided to the right, whereas two birds with wings spread (a small white dove and an owl) occupied the left. In front stood a Guan Yin figurine. Opposite to Guan Yin, in the lower left corner stood the Jesus figurine with his hands raised. A huge rainbow and a round-shaped stone were behind him.

In front of Jesus, many children, a newlywed couple, some teenagers and adults as well as two Native Americans on horses gathered beside a Christmas tree and a small golden tree. Two houses and a lighthouse as well as trees, shells, rocks, marbles were present in this area to the left.

On the land on the right hand side, outside of the animals mentioned above, other animals were: a group of pigs; deer; kangaroos; and butterflies. A huge selection of blossoming flowers (some were brought in by Jade), small trees, and fruit were also present.

At each of the two bridges, about to cross, were a man and a woman, each pushing a cart carrying watermelons. Two boats entered the river at the upper left and lower right corners, with one of the boats, a canoe carrying a Native American chief sitting behind an Native American male, headed toward the upper left direction.

Jade's comments

Jade said:

> This side [the right area] is very peaceful and serene; that side [the left area] is where your heart can be rested and trustful. These birds [upper right] are very carefree. Children here [left side] are protected by God. This couple comes here to make a promise, a covenant. The horse riders are very powerful. The bridges are for crossing; people can freely cross back and forth. The left side is a treasure land, shiny and full of power. I feel it is a covenant to me, a beautiful and an abundant place. I feel I have the strength to face future challenges; I do not have to fight them; instead, I can deal with them.
>
> About separation, I am not fearful, I can accept it. However, a small regret is that I still do not dare to grab the big snakes by hand. That will be the challenge in the future. In the sand tray, I see and find myself. I also

see the promise, the covenant, and I feel very steady and firm. Even though I may not know the nature of this accomplishment, I am most proud of facing the major challenge of my life. It is really worthwhile.

Therapist's interpretations

The severe depression and the splitting selves seen in the first tray made by Jade have been resolved. Jade's sand picture here shows the integration of polarity and a meaningful as well as free connection between the outer world and inner world with both being peaceful, serene, productive, protective, and blessed.

In this last sand tray, one can see the abundant life energy, represented by the Native Americans in the canoe and on horses, and by the wings-spread, ready-to-fly birds. Jade has found herself, and is, as she claimed, reborn; she has been in darkness and now she has found the light. This is truly a rebirth process.

Chapter 15

Summary

For every client, going through the sandplay process is not an easy task. It is often filled with obstacles, sometimes dangers, and at times, many challenges. Sandplay is a depth psychology; it deals with the unconscious, the shadowy side of oneself. Thus, every professional therapist who wishes to use this approach must first enter his or her own sandplay process. Then, he or she may learn that it is a highly powerful approach. It can be very constructive, and yet it has its destructive potential as well. The case of Jade illustrates the power of sandplay deeply and clearly.

In the beginning stage of this process, Jade immediately regressed. She became lost, severely depressed, and was highly polarized. The apparently relatively normal self was very threatened by the underdeveloped emotional self; thus, early suppressed suicidal ideas surfaced (Jade had periodic suicidal thoughts during her childhood as well as teenage years). Her depressive symptoms originated from her earlier distorted belief that "I am unwanted," or, "I do not belong in this family."

Due to the early crisis situation, I, as a therapist, was more active in enacting suicidal preventive strategies. Thus, there was more verbal therapy than sand tray creation. One can tell from Jade's early sand trays entitled "The me who is lost," "Who is or are under the tombstones?", "My tomb," and "Vast depression and a breathing oasis" (Figures 14.1 to 14.4) that Jade was lost and depressed, threatened by the unconscious materials.

Gradually, Jade was willing to enter the "Fantasy world" (Figure 14.5), encounter the "Fireworks of life" (Figure 14.6), and enter "The gate" (Figure 14.7) as well as the Safe Harbor (sand picture omitted) and the "The safe hideout" (Figure 14.8). The phenomenon of centering as defined by Weinrib became apparent. Jade, after making many more trays, reached the tray that was entitled "After all, I am not an unwanted child!" (Figure 14.13). That was a turning point. After that, she made several beautiful mandala trays in a row.

The "Tears" tray (Figure 14.15) came right after my taking a summer vacation that lasted two and a half months. Even though Jade denied the anger, she was briefly lost again and recovered shortly thereafter. Many trays that represented her healthy integration of splitting selves were made. Moreover, an abundant life energy bubbled which led to some brief periods of manic-like symptoms. Jade did numerous art projects to release these overly abundant energies. It was not until she gave me a gift of her art creation that she finally felt stabilized and in control.

During the last stage, separation anxiety took place. I used both verbal therapy and sandplay to help her deal with this anxiety. When Jade made the "Going toward the light" tray (Figure 14.22) in which a horse carriage is heading toward the distant rainbow, she and I knew the separation anxiety was gone and the end of our work was very near. Her last tray, "Rebirth" (Figure 14.24), clearly reflects her readiness to leave this process and to go on the rest of her life journey on her own.

In conclusion of this chapter, I would like, with her permission, to have Jade share her own story (translated from the Chinese by me) that was published in the newsletter of the Taiwanese Sandplay Therapy Association several years ago, a year before she finished the process.

> The sandplay process that has taken place in these three years turned out to be the most important experience of my life; it was incredibly rich and most wonderful. In these three years, I rapidly experienced many stages of my life, and a few times I almost could not make it through or endure. With Dr. Hong's persistent prayers, my faith in her, and most importantly her professionalism, I was able to overcome the cold, dark days. It was as if the withered trees flourished again in the springtime; I became alive. Presently, I am filled with courage and energy; there is a clear life goal. I am adventurous, willing to meet the challenges.
>
> There was, however, a lengthy period when I was very down, very anxious, having no desire to enter the sandplay room, and wanting to cancel appointments. Yet I knew if I did, I would hate myself so much, so I did not cancel. Entering the therapy room, feeling so heavy and down, I would start to complain about things in my life to Dr. Hong while eyeing the sand trays, telling them in my heart, "I don't want to be near you; I hate you; do not bother me; why are you there?" At that moment, they made me felt so frustrated and defeated.
>
> Not wanting to admit my defeat, I would reluctantly pick up miniatures and place them in a sand tray. Upon completion and examination of the tray, I would hate myself so much because I felt it was not what I wanted. Exiting the sandplay room, I began to tell myself, "What are you doing? Why are you wasting your time?"
>
> A month passed, a year passed, and nearly two years passed, I got worse. I was dissatisfied with any tray that I made, and I began to tell myself, "Why don't you just give up and kill yourself?" Right around that time, I seriously contemplated death. Every night my tears fell like rain from the sky, and I felt like I was experiencing a severe depression.

Dr. Hong's presence plus her support were the only light that I saw at that time.

One day after work, I was so down and could not endure my pain any longer. I thought I might as well step in front of a car and get it over with. I prayed to God, "What do you want me to do? I have a very elderly mother, a loving husband, and two wonderful children. What shall I do?" I pleaded with God, "Help me! Help me!" All of a sudden, a warm sensation started to grow from my heart, gradually spreading through my whole body. I felt love and supportive power all over. "Wow! Someone loves me!" I said to myself, beginning to cry. I was in tears all the way home. It was as if I were in my father's arms, crying about all the hurt that I had received in the past, and that he was cuddling me, embracing me, and telling me that he loves me. From that moment on, the protective theme appeared in my sand trays, and I knew that I had the strength to live.

For a short period, I thought the rain was gone and that I was all right. When Dr. Hong returned to Taiwan from the United States after her summer vacation for our first session, the same old anxious feeling was back. Looking at the sand tray, I could not find myself; I felt dreadful and was filled with extreme despair. Seeing the sand tray, the fire of anger arose from my feet. I was angry at myself, at everything, especially angry that I had given up so easily when faced with this difficulty. At that moment, Dr. Hong asked me, "Are you angry at me because I went to the US and was away for such a long time?" I angrily said in my heart, "Who are you? Why should I be angry at you? Are you that important to me?" My God, I truly collapsed. In order to not completely crumble, I pulled myself up, grabbed some miniatures, and told myself: "You know what you want. Whatever you take is what you want, now, I order you to take them!" I struggled and struggled. With my trembling hands, I put the miniatures, one by one, in the tray, telling myself: "This is what you want; this is truly what you want!" I used up all my energy and finished the tray.

Upon completion, I felt totally exhausted; my energy was completely spent. Nevertheless, I knew my energy would be back because I heard my voice—I truly heard my voice. The "I" was so strong and powerful. I finally met "I," the self. "I" was born; it is the most wonderful feeling I have ever experienced. I can feel; I can touch; I can hear; I can sense; everything is real; the fog is gone. In retrospect, I knew why I told Dr. Hong that I was not angry at her. At that time, I did not think anyone would care about me, and I did not dare to have that kind of expectation. Now I know I was wrong. Many people care about me, including Dr. Hong, of course.

From then on, I have never hesitated or wanted to avoid doing a sand tray; I know my hands will know what to take and how to do a tray that is according to what I really want. Based on every tray that I made, I was so pleased that I got to meet myself and to know myself; I treasure every tray that I made.

Sand tray has become my "other mother"; she trusted me, contained me, and gave me abundant love. In the sand tray, I found my "other mother," and I found the home for my soul.

Jade went on to talk about her separation anxiety in regards to leaving the sandplay process. As I noted before, we were able to deal with it, and Jade finished the sandplay process about a year after the above story which she wrote. To end this summary, I would like to share the final feedback that Jade wrote about the process:

> The best accomplishment about my sandplay process is that I became in touch with myself. Everything is real and firm. I can see; I can feel; and I can touch. To be in touch with the self is such a wonderful thing. The miracle has happened to me; the curse that was placed on the princess has been lifted. I am alive!

Appendix

I, Dr. Grace Hong, am invited to speak at the ISST Congress about my Taiwan sandplay experiences. Therefore, I would like to gather the information from those who have completed their sandplay processes. The information I am collecting is twofold, as shown below. Please take some time to fill out this form. You may choose to sign or not sign your name.

Sandplay therapy outcome survey

In the following areas, what positive impact has your sandplay experience had on you? Please check all that apply.

- ——Self-Concept/Image
- ——Emotional Stability
- ——Interpersonal Relationships
- ——Communication and Expressive Ability
- ——Cognitive and Logic Ability
- ——Objective Awareness of Events in Life
- ——Problem-Solving Ability
- ——Independence and Self-Assertion
- ——Frustration Tolerance
- ——Self-Confidence
- ——Psychological Energy
- ——Sense of Responsibility
- ——Physical Health
- ——Spiritual Growth

Other areas: _____ _____ _____ _____

Within one hundred words, please state your thoughts and feelings about completing the sandplay process.

References

Achenbach, T.M. (1991). *Manual for the Teacher's Report Form and 1991 profile.* Burlington, VT: Department of Psychiatry, University of Vermont.
Allan, J. (1988). *Inscapes of the child's world.* Dallas, TX: Spring.
Allan, J. and Berry, P. (1987). Sandplay. *Elementary School Guidance and Counselling,* 24(4): 300–306.
Allen, J. and Griffiths, J. (1979). *The book of the dragon.* Secaucus, NJ: Chartwell.
Ammann, R. (1991). *Healing and transformation in sandplay.* La Salle, IL: Open Court.
Baskin, H. and Baskin, L. (1985). *A book of dragon.* New York: Alfred A. Knopf.
Biedermann, H. (1989). *Dictionary of symbolism: Cultural icons and the meanings behind them.* New York: Penguin.
Blumberg, R. (1980). *The truth about dragons.* New York: Four Winds Press.
Bradway, K. (1987). Sandplay: What makes it work? In M.A. Mattoon (ed.) *Proceedings of the Tenth International Congress of Analytical Psychology.* Einsiedeln, Switzerland: Daimon Verlag.
Bradway, K. (1990). Development stages in children's sand worlds. In K. Bradway, K. Signell, G. Spare, C. Stewart, L. Stewart, and C. Thompson, *Sandplay studies: Origins, theory and practice* (2nd edn) (pp. 93–100). Boston, MA: Sigo Press.
Bradway, K. (1991). Transference and countertransference in sandplay therapy. *Journal of Sandplay Therapy,* 1(1), 25–43.
Bradway, K. (1992). Sandplay in preparing to die. *Journal of Sandplay Therapy,* 2(1), 16–36.
Bradway, K. and McCoard, B. (1997). *Sandplay: Silent workshop of the psyche.* London: Routledge.
Bradway, K. and McCoard, B. (2005). *Sandplay: Silent workshop of the psyche,* Chinese translation. Taiwan: Wu-Nan.
Caproni, P.M. and Martin, P. (1989). Sandplay: Window on the representational world. A projective adaptation of Lowenfeld's world technique. *Dissertation Abstracts International,* 49(11-A), 3305.
Carey, L. (1990). Sandplay with a troubled child. *Arts in Psychotherapy,* 17(3), 197–209.
Chinen, A.B. (1999). *Once upon a midlife: Classic stories and mythic tales to illuminate the middle years,* Chinese translation. Taiwan: Morning Star.
Christie, A. (1985). *Chinese mythology.* New York: Peter Bedrick.

Cooper, J.C. (1979). *An illustrated encyclopedia of traditional symbols*. New York: Thames & Hudson.
de Mello, A. (1985). *One minute wisdom*. New York: Doubleday.
de Vries, A. (1984). *Dictionary of symbols and imagery*. Amsterdam: Elsevier Science.
Dickinson, P. (1979). *The flight of dragons*. London: Pierrot.
Domenico, D. and Schubach, G. (1987). The Lowenfeld World Apparatus: A methodological contribution towards the study and the analysis of the sand tray play process. *Dissertation Abstracts International*, *48*(5-B), 1510.
Eastwood, P. (1999). Resonance on symbol papers. *Journal of Sandplay Therapy*, *VIII*(1), 15–20.
Edinger, E.F. (1985). *Anatomy of the psyche: Alchemical symbolism in psychotherapy*. La Salle, IL: Open Court.
Edinger, E.F. (1992). *Ego and archetype: Individuation and the religious function of the psyche*. Boston, MA: Shambhala.
Exner, J.E. (1986). *The Rorschach: A comprehensive system. Volume 1: Basic foundations*. New York: Wiley.
Exner, J.E. (1990). *A Rorschach work book for the comprehensive system* (3rd edn). Asheville, NC: Rorschach Workshops.
Exner, J.E. and Weiner, I.B. (1986). *The Rorschach: A comprehensive system. Volume 3: Assessment of children and adolescents*. New York: Wiley.
Fontana, D. (1994). *The secret language of symbols: A visual key to symbols and their meanings*. San Francisco, CA: Chronicle Books.
Friedman, H.S. and Mitchell, R.R. (1991). Dora Maria Kalff: Connections between life and work. *Journal of Sandplay Therapy*, *1*(1), 17–23.
Harding, M.E. (1973). *The "I" and the "not-I": A study in the development of consciousness*. Princeton, NJ: Princeton University Press.
Hodges, M. (1984). *Saint George and the dragon*. Boston, MA: Little, Brown.
Hong, G.H.H.L. (1994). The dragon as a symbol. Unpublished manuscript.
Huxley, F. (1992). *The dragon* (2nd edn). New York: Thames & Hudson.
Johnsgard, P. and Johnsgard, K. (1982). *Dragons and unicorns: A natural history*. New York: St. Martin's.
Jung, C.G. (1961). *Memories, dreams, reflections*. New York: Pantheon.
Jung, C.G. (1968). *The archetypes and the collective unconscious* (2nd edn). Princeton, NJ: Princeton University Press.
Kalff, D.M. (1980). *Sandplay: A psychotherapeutic approach to the psyche*. Boston, MA: Sigo Press.
Kalff, D.M. (1991). Introduction to sandplay therapy. *Journey of sandplay Therapy*, *1*(1), 7–15.
Kalff, D.M. (2003). *Sandplay: A psychotherapeutic approach to the psyche* (Sandplay Classics series). Cloverdale, CA: Temenos.
Kalff, M. (1993). Twenty points to be considered in the interpretation of a sandplay. *Journey of Sandplay Therapy*, *2*(2), 17–35.
Kawai, H. (1988). *The Japanese psyche: Major motifs in the fairy tales of Japan*. Dallas, TX: Spring.
Kiepenheuer, K. (1990). *Crossing the bridge*. La Salle, IL: Open Court.
Kovacs, M. (1979). *The Children Depression Inventory*. Pittsburgh, PA: University of Pittsburgh School of Medicine.
McGowen, T. (1981). *Encyclopedia of legendary creatures*. Chicago, IL: Rand McNally.

Matthews, B. (1986). *The herder symbol dictionary*. Wilmette, IL: Chiron.
Miller, C. and Boe, J. (1990). Tears into diamonds: Transformation of child psychic trauma through sandplay and storytelling. *Arts in Psychotherapy*, *17*(3), 247–257.
Mitchell, R.R. and Friedman, H.S. (1992). Sandplay: Overview of the first sixty years. *Journal of Sandplay Therapy*, *1*(2), 27–35.
Neumann, E. (1990). *The child* (R. Manheim, trans.). Boston, MA: Shambhala.
Reece, S. (1995). The mound as healing image in sandplay. *Journal of Sandplay Therapy*, *4*(2), 15–31.
Ryce-Menuhin, J. (1988). *The self in early childhood*. London: Free Association Books.
Segal, J. (1990). Sandplay: A validation study of sandplay as a projective technique. *Dissertation Abstracts International*, *51*(6-B), 3146–3147.
Stewart, C.T. (1990). The developmental psychology of sandplay. In K. Bradway, K. Signell, C. Stewart, L. Stewart, and C. Thompson, *Sandplay studies: Origins, theory and practice* (2nd edn) (pp. 39–92). Boston, MA: Sigo Press.
Strupp, H.H. (1973). *Psychotherapy: Clinical, research, and theoretical issues*. New York: Jason Aronson.
Vinturella, L. and James, R. (1987). Sandplay: A therapeutic medium with children. *Elementary School Guidance and Counseling*, *21*(3), 229–238.
Walker, B.G. (1988). *The woman's dictionary of symbols and sacred objects*. New York: HarperCollins.
Weinrib, E.L. (1983). *Images of the self: The sandplay therapy process*. Boston, MA: Sigo Press.
Weinrib, E.L. (2004). *Images of the self: The sandplay therapy process* (Sandplay Classic series). Cloverdale, CA: Temenos.
Weller, B. (1997). So you have to write a symbol paper! *Journal of Sandplay Therapy*, *VI*(1), 15–19.
Williams, C.A.S. (1976). *Outline of Chinese symbolism and art motives: Third revised edition with 402 illustrations*. New York: Dover.
Zappacosta, F.D. (1992). Healing our children: Divine energies in play. *Journal of Sandplay Therapy*, *2*(1), 59–65.

Index

alcohol abuse 59
alienation 56, 60, 64, 97, 98, 142;
    acceptance of alienated self 149
Allan, J. 20; and Berry, P. 20
Allen, J. and Griffiths, J. 108, 109, 111–12
Ammann, R. 17, 20
anger 32, 68, 89–90, 162, 182, 184
animals 66–7, 153, 174, 176, 177;
    see also specific animals
ants 62
Ashiao the fisherman story 106–7
assertion *see* self-assertion
attachment therapy 14

barrenness 42, 59, 62, 80, 97–8, 132, 144
Baskin, H. and Baskin, L. 110
Bayley, A. "Nessie" 13–14, 48
Bible 2–3, 58, 80, 109
birds 10, 66, 87, 128–9, 130, 154, 181;
    see also specific birds
black, color 68
black people and figures 57–8, 60, 63, 69, 71, 80, 81–2, 96, 163, 171
black identity 60, 72–3
Blumberg, R. 111
boats 92, 107, 127, 128, 154, 157, 158, 159, 167, 170, 173, 180
bottom-of-the-ocean scene 93
Bradway, K. 14–15, 18, 71, 103
bridge symbol 60, 71, 144, 153, 154
broomsticks 60
Buddha 93, 112, 127, 130, 147

caged bird 87
candles 153, 154, 163, 164
Carey, L. 20
carp 106, 107, 111

CDI (Children Depression Inventory) 24, 28–9, 51, 97
cedar wood 146, 147, 148, 149
centering 62, 71, 73, 83, 154, 172, 182; in mental health workers' sand pictures 122, 126, 127, 131
child archetype/symbol 59, 65, 87;
    mother-child unity (mother holding a baby) 147, 148, 152, 171, 175, 178
Child Protection Agency (US) 24, 44, 97
Children Depression Inventory (CDI) 24, 28–9, 51, 97
Chinen, A.B. 159, 167
clowns 149, 170, 171
co-transference 14–15, 72, 174
coffins 62
colors 66, 68; Rorschach coding and 32, 38, 39
coniunctio see union of opposites
connection symbols 60, 71, 144, 153, 154, 163, 167–8; *see also* boats
Cooper, J.C. 127
coral leaf 62
countertransference 14–15
courage 59, 60, 66, 80, 151
cross 80, 83–4, 92, 160, 161, 162
crown 87, 99

Daugherty, R. 13–14
de Mello, A. 105
de Vries, A. 72, 125, 159
death: suicide *see* suicide; symbols of 84, 112, 125, 149; Zana's sand picture "Total death" 88–90, 99
demons 78, 79
depression 2, 20, 68; Children Depression Inventory 24, 28–9, 51, 97; Jade case 146, 148, 156, 159, 182,

183–4; Rorschach morbid content coding 33–4
Dickinson, P. 108
donkey 66–7
Dorothy figure 75, 76, 88, 95, 98
doves, white 152, 153, 175, 176, 177, 178, 180
dragon king's daughter, myth of 9–10, 106–7
dragon symbol: author's study of 105–13; dragon poems 113; dragons in mythology, folklore, and religion 109–10; Eastern and Western dragons contrasted 110–11; horses and dragons 107–8, 109, 112; Jade case 149; question of one-time existence of dragons 108–9; slaying the dragon 111–12; Zana case 78–9, 112–13
dreams 78, 79, 103, 112–13; of the author 11; Jade case 143, 144, 175–6
Driscoll, R. 27, 41–2, 52
ducks 66, 70, 123, 131, 151, 154, 157, 173, 175

Eastwood, P. 103
Eden, Garden of 176, 179
Edinger, E.F. 60, 64, 69, 88–9
ego-Self 13; alienation 60, 64, 97; axis 60, 71, 98; old wise man as personification of 60
emotional representations: in House-Tree-Person drawings 42, 43; in painting 68; Rorschach codings 32, 33, 39
emptiness 45, 64–5, 74
energy 2, 18, 59, 133, 134, 135; archetypal 16; blocked 16; divine 20; House-Tree-Person drawings and 42, 43; instinctual 66; Jade case 145, 149, 157, 167, 170, 174, 177, 179, 181, 183, 184; symbols of 60, 87, 130, 131, 145, 149, 154, 179, 181; unconscious 134
enlightenment 65, 87
execution scene and ritual 92

fish-dragons 111
five, number 132, 159
flags 157
floor games 48
flowers 74, 94, 121, 126–7, 128, 130, 131, 132; Jade case study 142, 143, 144, 145–6, 149, 150, 152, 158, 160, 162, 163, 167, 168, 171, 173, 174, 175, 178, 180; lotus 93
four, number 94, 109, 122, 132, 159, 164, 167
freedom 152–3, 174
frogs 143, 144, 168
fruitfulness 2, 123, 129

Garden of Hope Foundation, Taiwan 117
ghosts 61, 62, 149
golden key and the dragon king's daughter myth 9–10
golden throne 74, 86, 87, 99
graveyards 143, 144, 145, 159
green, colour 65, 68
Greenberg, L. 21, 23
ground symbolism 83
Guan Yin figure 121, 128, 171, 172, 180

H-T-P (House-Tree-Person) drawings 24, 27, 41–3, 51, 52
Harding, M.E. 87
Hodges, M. 110
Hong, Minna 113
horses, dragons and 107–8, 109, 112
House-Tree-Person (H-T-P) drawings 24, 27, 41–3, 51, 52
Hutchinson, J. 26–7, 37–9, 52
Huxley, F. 107, 110

immortality 2, 60, 65, 66, 93, 109, 112, 125
innocence 59; lost 59, 90
integration 10, 16; Jade case study 142–3, 144, 146, 159, 163, 164, 167–8, 176, 181, 183; of masculinity and femininity 69, 85, 94, 95, 98–9; Rorschach coding and 38, 39; Zana case study 60, 71, 80, 85, 95, 98–9; *see also* union of opposites
International Society for Sandplay Therapy (ISTG) 1, 7, 18–19, 103
islands 158–9, 166–9

Jade case study *see* sandplay therapy case study, Jade
Jesus figure 83, 128, 162, 163, 164, 180
Johnsgard, P. and Johnsgard, K. 108
Jung, C.G. 12, 59, 60, 85, 112, 159

Kalff, D.M. 12–13, 18, 19, 73, 164
Kalff, M. 15

Kawai, H. 15, 16–17, 118
Kendall Self-Rating Scale 21, 23
Kiepenheuer, K. 20
Kinetic Family Drawing 56
Kukulcan 109

ladders 60
lakes 9–10, 92, 153, 159, 162, 178, 179
lamps 65
lion 66
loneliness 168–9
lotus 93

McGowan, T. 111
mandala 93, 94, 163–4, 165, 172
marbles 76, 77, 93, 94, 96, 98, 132, 165, 166
Mary figure (St Mary) 164, 167, 168, 171, 172, 175, 176, 178
Miller, C. and Boe, J. 20
Minneapolis research study *see* sandplay therapy research study, Minneapolis
Minnesota Sandplay Therapy Group (MSTG) 7, 21, 23, 25, 74
mirrors 74, 87
moon 62
mother-child unity (mother holding a baby) 147, 148, 152, 171, 175, 178
mountains 153, 154; mountain village 175–6
mourning 59

National Taiwan University 8
Native American figures 91–2, 162–3, 164, 167, 168, 171, 177, 180, 181; mother holding a baby 147, 148
negative transference 142, 166
Neumann, E. 18
neurosis, alienation 64
numerical symbolism 83, 94, 122, 132, 159, 164, 167
nuns 164, 171, 172

oak tree 59, 80, 132
old wise man archetype 60
owls 128, 174

paint pictures 67–8, 88–9, 94
passivity 64, 97; Rorschach coding 35
peacock 66
phallic symbolism 88
pine tree 65

pipe cleaners 150, 151, 152
polar bear 80
pots 65
prayer 148, 183, 184; praying hands 125, 162
preacher figure 58, 60, 80
priest figure 83, 160, 162, 164
prima materia 92, 112
Primal Waters 111
protection 149, 170, 172, 181, 184; divine 125, 128, 129, 136, 180; need for 59, 97; protective symbols 59, 92, 121, 123, 128, 129, 130, 146, 148, 149–50, 162, 163, 167, 168, 172, 179; strategies of 139; therapy's protective space 9, 13, 15, 17, 133, 134, 135, 136
psychotherapy outcome research 21–2
pyramids 125

Quetzalcoatl 109

rainbows 60, 88, 128, 155, 156
rebirth 18, 62, 69, 87, 90, 97–8; Jade's sandplay rebirth process 141–81, 182–5; in mental health workers' sand pictures 127, 131–3; *see also* regeneration
reconciliation 80, 94
red 68
redemption 62, 84
regeneration 121, 125, 127, 131, 132, 133; *see also* rebirth
rockets 149
Rorschach (Exner method) 24, 26, 29–39, 51, 52; Zana case study 56, 97
roses 150
Ryce-Menuhin, J. 20

sacred place 74
sadness 17, 43, 68, 89
sandplay therapist training 103
sandplay therapy case study, Jade: introduction of the case 139–40; sandplay rebirth process 141–81; summary 182–5
sandplay therapy case study, Zana: and the dragon symbol 78–9, 112–13; introduction of the case 55–6; paint pictures 67–8, 88–9, 94; sandplay process and recovery from sexual trauma 57–96, 97–100; summary 97–100

sandplay therapy literature: history of sandplay therapy 12–19; psychotherapy outcome research 21–2; sandplay therapy outcome research 19–21
sandplay therapy process 9–11
sandplay therapy research study, Minneapolis: Children Depression Inventory 28–9; conclusion 51–2; House-Tree-Person drawings 41–3; location 23; method 23–7; recommendations for future research 49–50; results and discussion 28–50; Rorschach 29–39; scoring of the tests 26–7; study limitations 47–9; subjects 23–4; Teacher's Report Form 39–41; therapists 25–6; therapists' reports 43–7
sandplay therapy research study, Taiwan: final sand pictures and themes of each subject 120–33; introduction concerning author's teaching experiences 117–19; outcome study of twelve mental health workers 120–36; survey questions 186; survey results 133–6
Santa Claus 71, 72
self-assertion 44, 47, 98, 133, 134; Zana case 69, 73, 77, 98, 99
Self-Perception Profile for Children 21, 23
Self/self: acceptance of alienated self 149; being in touch with the self 185; ego-Self *see* ego-Self; manifestation of the Self 13, 73, 93, 98, 164; polarity of self 142, 169, 170; the reborn self 184; Self tray 96, 164, 172; transformation *see* self-transformation
self-transformation 134–6; Jade case study 144; Zana case study 62, 66, 71–2, 84, 92, 93, 98–9; *see also* rebirth; regeneration
separation anxiety 183, 185
serenity 2, 123, 126, 129, 130, 131, 132
sexual trauma, sandplay and recovery from 57–96, 97–100
shadow 18, 79, 98, 134, 144, 176
Shen Lung 110
snakes 121, 136, 160, 161, 167, 174, 180; and the dragon of mythology 109
soul 17; journey 62, 64–5, 77, 98
spider webs 62

split selves 142, 169, 170
starfish 89, 143, 144, 162
Stewart, C.T. 17–18
Strupp, H.H. 21–2, 47, 48
sublimatio symbolism 88–9
suicide: Children Depression Inventory and 28, 29, 51; Jade's suicidal tendencies 139, 145, 146, 155, 161, 182, 183; Rorschach coding and 32, 33–4
Sun Wu-Kong 112
swans 66, 89, 131, 143, 144
swimming 143, 144
symbols 9–10; animal 66–7 *see also specific animals and birds*; of connection and communication 60, 71, 144, 153, 154, 163, 167–8 *see also* boats; of courage 59, 66, 80, 151; of death 84, 112, 125, 149; dragon symbol *see* dragon symbol; of emotions 68; of energy 60, 87, 130, 131, 145, 149, 154, 179, 181, 184; of freedom 152–3; of immortality 60, 65, 66, 93, 109, 112, 125; importance in sandplay therapy 103–4; numeric 83, 94, 122, 132, 159, 164, 167; phallic clay work 88; protective 59, 92, 121, 123, 128, 129, 130, 146, 148, 149–50, 162, 163, 167, 168, 172, 179; stages in studying a symbol 103; *sublimatio* symbolism 88–9; of wholeness 59, 66, 83, 94, 132, 164, 167, 172; *see also specific symbols and figures*
synchronicity 78, 107–8, 134

Taiwanese Sandplay Therapy Association 1, 183
Teacher's Report Form (TRF) 24, 39–41, 51
tears 90, 147, 165, 166, 183
throne, golden 74, 86, 87, 99
Thunder God 110
touch therapy 14
transcendence 84
transcendental function 71
transference 14–15; co-transference 14–15, 72, 174; negative 142, 166; Zana case 66, 69
transformation *see* self-transformation
the transpersonal 18
trees 80, 125, 131, 132; cutting down of 89; H-T-P drawings *see* House-Tree-Person (H-T-P) drawings; oak 59, 80,

132; pine 65; sea tree of Mother Goddess 62
TRF (Teacher's Report Form) 24, 39–41, 51
the unconscious 142–3; and the dragon symbol 111–12; and the history of sandplay therapy 12–13; the shadow (personal unconscious) 18, 79, 98, 144, 176; symbols and the conflict between the conscious and 9–10

union of opposites 59–60, 71, 82, 85, 87; integration/union of masculinity and femininity 69, 85, 94, 95, 98–9; Jade case 167–8, 172; *see also* integration

Vinturella, L. and James, R. 20

Wagstaff, A. 7
water 66, 69, 89–90, 131; and the dragon king's daughter myth 9–10; Primal Waters 111; and swimming 143, 144
wedding picture 82
Weinrib, E.L. 15–16, 18, 19–20, 154
Weller, B. 7, 26, 48, 103, 117
whale 143, 144
white doves 152, 153, 175, 176, 177, 178, 180
wholeness 2, 13, 122, 131, 133, 167; symbols of 59, 66, 83, 94, 132, 164, 167, 172; Zana case 59, 60, 62, 66, 83, 84, 94, 97
Wiersma, J. 7, 117
Williams, C.A.S. 110–11
wisdom 60, 74, 78, 159, 174
wise old man archetype 60
witches 62, 170, 172, 174

Year of the Dragon 105, 106, 107
Yin and Yang 143, 159, 167–8
Yoda figure 62, 95

Zana case study *see* sandplay therapy case study, Zana
Zappacosta, F.D. 20